Intraoperative Graft Patency Verification in Cardiac and Vascular Surgery

edited by

Giuseppe D'Ancona, MD
Division of Cardiothoracic Surgery
State University of New York at Buffalo Buffalo, New York

Hratch L. Karamanoukian, MD
Clinical Assistant Professor of Surgery
Division of Cardiothoracic Surgery
State University of New York at Buffalo;
Associate Director
Center for Less Invasive Cardiac Surgery
and Robotic Heart Surgery
Buffalo General Hospital, Buffalo, New York

Marco Ricci, MD, PhD
Division of Cardiothoracic Surgery
University of Miami/Jackson Memorial Hospital
Miami, Florida

Tomas A. Salerno, MD
Professor and Chief
Division of Cardiothoracic Surgery
University of Miami/Jackson Memorial Hospital, Miami, Florida

Jacob Bergsland, MD
Clinical Associate Professor of Surgery
Division of Cardiothoracic Surgery
State University of New York Buffalo;
Director
Center for Less Invasive Cardiac Surgery
and Robotic Heart Surgery
Buffalo General Hospital
Buffalo, New York

Futura Publishing Company, Inc
Armonk, NY

Library of Congress Cataloging-in-Publication Data

Intraoperative graft patency verification in cardiac and vascular surgery /
edited by Giuseppe D'Ancona . . . [et al.].
    p.; cm.
  Includes bibliographical references and index.
  ISBN 0-87993-488-3 (alk. paper)
    1. Coronary artery bypass. 2. Vascular grafts. 3. Blood flow. 4. Coronary heart disease. 5. Heart-Surgery. I. D'Ancona, Giuseppe.
    [DNLM: 1. Coronary Artery Bypass. 2. Blood Flow Velocity—physiology. 3. Cardiac Surgical Procedures. 4. Graft Occlusion, Vascular—surgery. WG 169 G737 2001]
RD598.35.C67 G73 2001
617.4'1—dc21

                                  2001018934

Copyright 2001
Futura Publishing Company, Inc.

Published by
Futura Publishing Company
135 Bedford Road
Armonk, New York 10504
www.futuraco.com

LC#: 2001018934
ISBN#: 0-87993-488-3

*To all of the colleagues and friends
who have contributed to the
realization of this book.*

Contributors

Guido Beldi, MD
Cardiovascular Surgery Department, University Hospital Inselspital, Bern, Switzerland

Jacob Bergsland, MD
Clinical Associate Professor of Surgery, Division of Cardiothoracic Surgery, State University of New York Buffalo; Director, Center for Less Invasive Cardiac Surgery, and Robotic Heart Surgery, Buffalo General Hospital, Buffalo, New York

Andreas Bosshard, MD
Cardiovascular Surgery Department, University Hospital Inselspital, Bern, Switzerland

Carlos E. Brockmann, MD
Cardiovascular Surgeon, Departments of Cardiovascular and Thoracic Surgery, Cardiology, and Biostatistics, University Clinics (Université Catholique de Louvain), of Mont Godinne, Yvoir, Belgium

Thierry Carrel, MD
Professor of Cardiovascular Surgery, Cardiovascular Surgery Department, University Hospital Inselspital, Bern, Switzerland

Patricia B. Cerrito, PhD
Professor of Mathematics and Biostatistician, Jewish Hospital Heart and Lung Institute, University of Louisville, Louisville, Kentucky

Giuseppe D'Ancona, MD
Division of Cardiothoracic Surgery, State University of New York at Buffalo, Buffalo, New York

Gabriele Di Giammarco, MD
Division of Cardiac Surgery, San Camillo de Lellis Hospital, Chieti, Italy

Harry W. Donias, M.D.
General Surgery Resident, Department of Surgery, State University of New York at Buffalo, Buffalo, New York

Erik Fosse, MD
The Interventional Centre, Rikshospitalet, Oslo, Norway

Olivier Gurné, MD, PhD
Cardiologist, Departments of Cardiovascular and Thoracic Surgery, Cardiology, and Biostatistics, University Clinics (Université Catholique de Louvain) of Mont Godinne, Yvoir, Belgium

Otto M. Hess, MD
Professor of Cardiology, Cardiovascular Surgery Department, University Hospital Inselspital, Bern, Switzerland

Per Kristian Hol, MD
The Interventional Centre, Rikshospitalet, Oslo, Norway

Jacques Jamart, MD
Biostastician, Departments of Cardiovascular and Thoracic Surgery, Cardiology, and Biostatistics, University Clinics (Université Catholique de Louvain) of Mont Godinne, Yvoir, Belgium

Hratch L. Karamanoukian, MD
Clinical Assistant Professor of Surgery, Division of Cardiothoracic Surgery, State University of New York at Buffalo; Associate Director, Center for Less Invasive Cardiac Surgery, and Robotic Heart Surgery, Buffalo General Hospital, Buffalo, New York

Steven C. Koenig, PhD
Assistant Professor of Surgery, Jewish Hospital Cardiothoracic Surgical Research Institute at the University of Louisville, Department of Surgery, University of Louisville, Louisville, Kentucky

Jesper Laustsen, MD
Chief Vascular Surgeon, Department of Cardiothoracic and Vascular Surgery and Institute of Experimental Clinical Research, Aarhus University Hospital, Aarhus, Denmark

Yves A.G. Louagie, PhD, MD
Professor, Cardiovascular and Thoracic Surgeon, Departments of Cardiovascular and Thoracic Surgery, Cardiology and Biostatistics, University Clinics (Université Catholique de Louvain) of Mont Godinne, Yvoir, Belgium

Anders Lundell, MD, PhD
Department of Vascular Diseases, Malmo/Lund, Malmo University Hospital, Malmo, Sweden

Marco Ricci, MD, PhD
Division of Cardiothoracic Surgery, University of Miami/Jackson Memorial Hospital, Miami, Florida

Tomas A. Salerno, MD
Professor and Chief, Division of Cardiothoracic Surgery, University of Miami/Jackson Memorial Hospital, Miami, Florida

Susan Schmid, RN, RNFA
Clinical Coordinator, Minimally Invasive Cardiac Surgery, Kaleida Health, Buffalo General Division, Buffalo, New York

Paul A. Spence, MD
Professor of Surgery, Jewish Hospital Cardiothoracic Surgical Research Institute at the University of Louisville, Department of Surgery, University of Louisville, Louisville, Kentucky

Giuseppe Speziale, MD
Staff Surgeon, Department of Thoracic and Cardiovascular Surgery, Villa Azzurra Rapallo, Genova, Italy

Einar Stranden, PhD
Professor, Department of Vascular Diagnosis and Research, Aker Hospital, University of Oslo, Oslo, Norway

Beat H. Walpoth, MD
Cardiovascular Surgery Department, University Hospital Inselspital, Bern, Switzerland

Introduction

Quality assurance is a buzz phrase in modern medicine, and in most other types of human activity. According to Webster's Dictionary, quality assurance means *"a program for the systematic monitoring and evaluation of the various aspects of a project, service, or facility to ensure that standards of quality are being met."*

Quality assurance interfaces with many aspects of the cardiac surgeon's activity. Hospitals, insurers, government bodies, and health care organizations monitor results of what a cardiac surgeon does on an ongoing basis to define mortality and morbidity in defined groups of patients, and they monitor adverse outcomes in individual patients. Implantable devices and disposable material undergo rigorous testing by industry prior to FDA approval and actual use in patients.

The surgical procedure and its result have often been less systematically evaluated for quality assurance. Many aspects of surgical procedures are still considered part of the art rather than the science of surgery, and because of this there may be extreme controversies about who and what is a good surgeon from a technical point of view. Most practitioners of the art of surgery still recognize the need for some kind of quality assurance tool in their different surgical activities, not only a count of dead and live bodies but a documentation of the fact that what they did actually worked. We frequently hear statements such as, "I did a perfect job," "that was a beautiful anastomosis," etc. In most procedures, we would like to see some proof that the intended result of the procedure was accomplished. After a chest tube insertion, most of us order a chest x-ray to satisfy ourselves, the patient, the quality assurance committee, and potential lawyers that the tube is actually in the chest. We do a quick and slick pacemaker insertion, but we also want to measure the pacing threshold and see the lead position on fluoroscopy. After we have done "a beautiful valve repair," most of us prefer something more than visual admiration, namely a quantifiable picture on transesophageal echo (TEE). Even on a straightforward aortic valve replacement, most of us probably like to see a TEE to make sure that our perfect suturing was really perfect. When using cold cardioplegia, some of us measure myocardial temperature rather than trusting that the "heart feels pretty cold."

How do we assure quality in coronary bypass surgery? It seems to be a paradox that when we realize the need to demonstrate that our procedures work in most of our daily tasks, coronary anastomosis has been left out. In no area of the cardiac surgeon's activity has self-admiration and unproven confidence been more prevalent than in the performance of the coronary anastomosis. There may be multiple explanations for this confidence. First of all, standard coronary artery bypass grafting (CABG) has become a highly reliable procedure with overall low mortality rates and documented long-term benefits. The best surgeons in the country have reported graft patencies in the 90% range, and of course everyone assumes that their graft patency was the same if they used a technique similar to the published results. Second, the tools available to assure properly functioning grafts are rather cumbersome. Electromagnetic flow measurements are quite complex and somewhat unreliable and need constant calibration. Intraoperative angiography requires expensive equipment in the operating room and availability of invasive cardiologists. Angiography also has significant potential for adverse effects, particularly due to the need for injection of contrast material. Simple Doppler probes can demonstrate the presence of flow in the graft but without easy quantification of flow.

When we embarked on off-pump bypass surgery in Buffalo in 1995, graft patency was definitely a major concern. We were operating on a moving heart without mechanical stabilization in a relatively hostile environment. It was a humbling experience in the early phase. Each time we finished a graft, we would wonder: is that graft really patent? Honestly, we believe that the more self-critical of us always asked this question despite the type of cardiopulmonary bypass technique used, because there is no doubt that coronary artery surgery is difficult and requires excellent manual skills, and life and death issues are riding on very small technical details. When we started to work on the beating heart, the need to verify patency of the grafts became a major priority for our team.

We soon started to utilize transit time flow measurement (TTFM) as a quality assurance tool and we demonstrated quickly that a number of grafts needed revision due to technical reasons. TTFM was highly reliable in the detection of obstructed grafts. TTFM was very simple to use, truly minimally invasive, and inexpensive. As more sophisticated devices became available, it was possible to further evaluate the characteristics of the graft flows and possibly refine the criteria for a good graft.

The study of coronary anatomy and physiology is a complex science. The ultimate goal of reconstructive vascular or coronary surgery is to have an anatomically perfect anastomosis, which supplies adequate flow to the tissues at rest and during exercise. How do we confirm that this is the case? In the preoperative phase, we usually utilize both a physiological test such as a stress test and an anatomical test such as the angiogram.

The interventionist uses at least an anatomical test such as an angiogram after the application of an intravascular device. Intravascular ultrasound is also a useful technique. Intravascular flow or pressure measurements may provide crucial physiological data when the anatomical situation is unclear. This book tries to answer certain important questions for the surgeon involved in vascular surgery whether it applies to the heart, the peripheral vascular system, or even organ transplantation.

Dr. Harry Donias' opening chapter gives an overview of basic rheology as it applies to the vascular system. He reintroduces the reader to basic concepts as they relate to blood flow.

Dr. Einar Stranden's chapter gives a comprehensive review of clinical methodology available for functional and anatomical testing of graft patency in vascular surgery.

An overview of the TTFM methodology applied clinically is outlined by Dr. Jesper Laustsen.

Dr. Anders Lundell gives an extensive review of flow measurements used in a variety of clinical settings in vascular and general surgery. He describes the pitfalls and drawbacks of different methods of flow measurements.

One of the major difficulties in the utilization of flow measurements in coronary surgery is the highly variable absolute flow values depending on a multitude of factors. Dr. Giuseppe Speziale gives an in-depth discussion of competitive flow and steal phenomena in coronary surgery. This chapter is crucial for the understanding of graft verification using TTFM.

Dr. Giuseppe D'Ancona describes the Buffalo Experience with TTFM in coronary surgery, which may be the largest experience in the world to date.

The group in Chieti, Italy, has extensive experience with TTFM used in a large series of minimally invasive and off-pump CABG surgeries. Dr. Gabriele Di Giammarco elegantly analyzes this experience.

One of the greatest challenges in TTFM interpretation is to reliably predict less than critical stenosis in the grafts or anastomosis. This has been demonstrated to be difficult to do by visual analysis. Dr. Paul Spence's group in Louisville has described one of the interesting approaches to this problem. Their automated classification system and neural network model may well be a valuable approach for a more comprehensive graft evaluation.

Dr. Erik Fosse, who is working at a fully equipped interventional center in Oslo, Norway, has used a combination of anatomical and physiological methods in studying his coronary bypass patients. Although this approach may be considered ideal, it may be very difficult to utilize in hospitals focused on "production" with high-volume clinical material. Since the ultimate goal is to establish adequate flow to the end organ, maybe measurement of flow makes the most sense as a quality assurance tool. However, flow measurements can be very difficult to evaluate, especially in the cardiac setting. As mentioned above, the purpose of this book is to attempt to answer some of the questions relating to graft verification in the clinical setting.

Dr. Yves Louagie has carefully analyzed the predictive value of Doppler on postoperative patency of bypass grafts. His chapter significantly contributes to the understanding of the value and limitations of TTFM.

Dr. Beat Walpoth is one of the pioneers in TTFM application to coronary surgery. In his chapter, he carefully compares different TTFM devices as well as gives valuable insight in how to apply the TTFM technique in cardiac surgery.

The last section of the book, the Appendix, is dedicated to practical examples of TTFM measurements from the large experience at Buffalo General Hospital. The examples were collected by Susan Schmid, RN, and will greatly assist new users of a TTFM device.

We believe that graft verification is a crucial aspect of quality assurance in coronary surgery. As we are moving toward totally endoscopic coronary bypass surgical procedures in the foreseeable future, demonstration of graft patency will be even more important. It is our hope that the readers of this book will benefit and take advantage of available technology for graft verification. Many of the complications seen in coronary surgery today are still due to poor graft function. If coronary surgery is to remain as a major clinical modality in the treatment of coronary artery disease, assurance of graft patency at the time of surgery is of critical importance.

Giuseppe D'Ancona, MD
Hratch L. Karamanoukian, MD
Marco Ricci, MD
Tomas A. Salerno, MD
Jacob Bergsland, MD

Contents

❖❖❖❖❖❖❖

❖❖❖❖❖❖

1

Rheology:

The Physical Basis of Blood Flow

Harry W. Donias, MD, Giuseppe D'Ancona, MD,
Hratch L. Karamanoukian, MD

Introduction

Luminal narrowing or occlusion of large arteries through the development of atherosclerotic plaque is the leading cause of death in the form of heart failure or stroke in the developed world.[1] Atherosclerosis is associated with genetic predisposition and multiple risk factors, including smoking, hypertension, diabetes mellitus, hyperlipidemia, sedentary lifestyle, and social stress. However, despite the systemic nature of its associated risk factors, atherosclerosis is a geometrically focal disease that commonly affects the artery only at certain well-defined locations rather than through its entire course.[2,3] Thus, it is strongly suspected that arterial hemodynamics play an important role in the genesis, progression, and regression of atherosclerosis.[1]

To understand the effects of hemodynamics on vascular diseases, it is necessary to review the physical nature of blood flow, also known as *rheology*. Blood flow in living organisms is complex and is influenced by many factors. In an attempt to describe quantitatively the flow of blood and its determinants, principles of fluid mechanics must be drawn upon. The equations most commonly used to describe blood flow, however, apply to the idealized case of nonpulsatile, laminar flow of homogeneous, Newtonian fluids in long, cylindrical tubes with rigid walls and were developed many years ago. In reality, rheology is not so simple, and therefore these equations are approximations at best. Nonetheless, keeping in

From: D'Ancona G, Karamanoukian HL, Ricci M, Salerno TA, Bergsland J (eds). *Intraoperative Graft Patency Verification in Cardiac and Vascular Surgery.* © Futura Publishing Company, Armonk, NY, 2001.

mind their limitations, they can be extremely useful in understanding many of the factors determining flow and how it is altered by various pathological states.[4] This chapter serves as a review of the basic equations and principles of rheology.

Total Hydraulic Energy

Total hydraulic energy (E) represents the sum of all forces contributing to the movement of fluid. For the purposes of this chapter, the fluid of interest is blood moving within the vascular system. In this model, blood moves from one point to another in the circulatory system in response to differences in total hydraulic energy.[5] The hydraulic energy associated with blood flow is of 2 kinds. The first is a potential energy (PE) that is manifested by blood pressure and is stored in the walls of the blood vessels on which that pressure acts.[6] The second kind is kinetic energy (KE).

$$E = PE + KE \qquad \text{[equation 1]}$$

The potential energy component is made up of intravascular pressure (P) and gravitational potential energy (ρgh).

$$PE = P + \rho gh \qquad \text{[equation 2]}$$

P is the sum of pressures produced by contraction of the heart (dynamic pressure), the hydrostatic pressure, and the static filling pressure of the resting circulation.[5]

$$P = P_{dynamic} + P_{hydrostatic} + P \qquad \text{[equation 3]}$$

Hydrostatic pressure results from the pressure produced by the weight of the fluid. In any body of water, the pressure at the surface of the water is equal to atmospheric pressure, but the pressure rises 1 millimeter of mercury (mm Hg) for each 13.6 mm distance below the surface due to the weight of the water. The same is true for the human vascular system, where the reference level for pressure measurement is the tricuspid valve. This is the point in the circulatory system at which hydrostatic pressure factors caused by changes in body position of a normal person usually do not affect the pressure measurement by more than 1 to 2 mm Hg.[7] The hydrostatic pressure in the vascular system is proportional to the weight of blood and is given by:

$$P_{hydrostatic} = -\rho gh \qquad \text{[equation 4]}$$

where ρ is the density of blood (approximately 1.056 gm/cm^3), g is the acceleration due to gravity (980 cm/sec^2), and h is the distance in centimeters from the reference level. It is important to remember that when one is talking about intravascular pressure, it generally means that this is at the hydrostatic level of the heart, but not necessarily elsewhere in the circulatory system, as this can be much higher for arteries farther away, such as in the feet.

The static filling pressure is related to the interaction between the elasticity of the vascular walls and the volume of blood contained within. This pressure is low, usually about 7 mm Hg in the human circulatory system.[5]

Gravitational potential energy represents the ability of a volume of blood to do work because of its elevation above the given reference point (the tricuspid valve). It is calculated in the same way as for hydrostatic pressure, but has an opposite sign ($+ \rho gh$).

$$PE_{gravitational} = + \rho gh \qquad \text{[equation 5]}$$

In many, but not all circumstances, gravitational potential energy and hydrostatic pressure will cancel each other out.[5]

The second kind of energy contributing to total hydraulic energy is kinetic energy, which represents the ability of blood to do work because of its motion.[5] It can be calculated from the physical mass of blood and the square of its velocity.[6]

$$KE = \tfrac{1}{2}\rho v^2 \qquad \text{[equation 6]}$$

where v refers to the velocity of a particle of blood moving in a straight line.

By substituting the above components into equation 1, the total hydraulic energy per unit volume of blood can be given by:

$$E = P + \rho gh + \tfrac{1}{2}\rho v^2 \qquad \text{[equation 7]}$$

where E is expressed in ergs per cubic centimeter.[5]

Bernoulli's Law

Bernoulli described the interaction of pressure, potential energy, and kinetic energy in the physics of flow in tubes. He used the equation for total hydraulic energy (equation 7) to demonstrate the conservation of energy in flowing fluids.[8] Bernoulli's law states that when fluid flows steadily (without acceleration or deceleration) from one point in a system to another farther downstream, its total energy content along any given streamline remains constant, provided there are no frictional losses.[5]

$$E = P_1 + \rho gh_1 + 1/2\rho v_1^2 = P_2 + \rho gh_2 + 1/2\rho v_2^2 \qquad \text{[equation 8]}$$

so that if the velocity should decrease downstream, total energy can be conserved by increasing the pressure. Likewise, if pressure decreases, total energy is conserved by increasing velocity. This is seen in the human body. As blood moves through the arterial tree, traversing the aorta, its larger primary branches, the smaller secondary branches, and the arterioles, the total vascular cross-sectional area gradually increases, and the velocity decreases. Finally, at the capillaries, the velocity decreases to a minimal value. All along this path the loss of kinetic energy, as a result of the loss of velocity, is partially converted into intravascular pressure to maintain the total energy. As the blood then passes through the venules and continues centrally toward the venae cavae, the velocity and the kinetic energy progressively increase at the expense of intravascular pressure.[6,9]

Bernoulli's principle also accounts for the pressure differences seen at different levels of the body. For example, when the pressure is measured at the feet of a standing person, it can be as much as 90 mm Hg higher than the pressure measured at the reference level. This is explained by the loss of gravitational potential energy that is converted to intravascular pressure as blood moves toward the feet. At levels progressively higher toward the reference level, the gravitational potential energy is again increased by increasing the height of the column of blood, and intravascular pressure decreases to maintain the total hydraulic energy.

Bernoulli's law applies only to an ideal Newtonian fluid moving along a streamline in a frictionless system. These conditions are never met in the human vascular system, or in any other real fluid system. However, the relationship between intravascular pressure, gravitational potential energy, and kinetic energy offers some explanation to the hemodynamics of the human body, and has been used since the relationship was established by Bernoulli in the 18th century.[8]

Velocity of the Bloodstream

Velocity refers to the rate of displacement of fluid with respect to time, and is expressed in units of distance per unit time (cm/sec). Flow, which is frequently called volume flow, is expressed in units of volume per unit time (cm^3/sec). In a tube with varying cross-sectional dimensions, velocity (v), flow (Q), and cross-sectional area (A) are related by the equation:

$$v = \frac{Q}{A} \qquad \text{[equation 9]}$$

The principle of conservation of mass requires that the flow of an incompressible fluid past successive cross-sections of a rigid tube must be constant.[9] For example, for a given simple tube with a cross-sectional area of 2 cm^2 and a velocity of 5 cm/sec, the flow would equal 10 cm^3/sec. If there was a segment of that tube where the area decreased to 1 cm^2, the velocity would increase to 10 cm/sec to maintain a flow of 10 cm^3/sec. If, for the same system, the cross-sectional area was increased to 5 cm^2, the velocity would have to decrease to 2 cm/sec to maintain a flow of 10 cm^3/sec.

In the arterial system, the arteries are not simple tubes, but have other arteries branching from them. If branch points are added to an artery, the total flow through the entire system remains constant, but the flow from the proximal artery to the distal end is reduced as a portion of the flow moves away from the parent vessel through the branching vessels. This can be seen in the coronary arterial system, where volume flow and daughter vessel cross-sectional area decrease from proximal to distal locations with branching, but velocity remains relatively preserved.[10]

The velocity of the fluid at any point in the system depends not only on the area, but also on the flow. Flow, in turn, depends on the pressure gradient, properties of the fluid, and dimensions of the entire hydraulic system. For any given flow, however, the ratio of the velocity past one cross-section relative to that past a second cross-section depends only on the inverse ratio of the respective areas,[9] thus:

$$\frac{v_1}{v_2} = \frac{A_2}{A_1} \qquad \text{[equation 10]}$$

Studies have shown that coronary flow velocity parameters are maintained across the normal epicardial artery so that velocity parameters in the distal segments do not differ significantly from those in the proximal segments. In contrast, volumetric flow diminishes along the vessel from proximal to distal segments, primarily because of the gradual reduction in epicardial vessel cross-sectional area, with total arterial perfusion area increased by branch vessels.[11] An example of this can be seen in Figure 1.

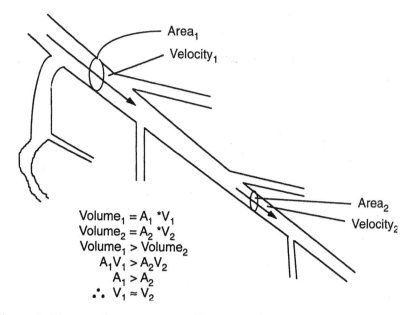

Figure 1. Diagram of coronary artery illustrating that coronary arteries normally branch frequently, that volumetric flow is proportional to velocity and cross-sectional area, and that as vessels taper, both cross-sectional area and volumetric flow are reduced, while velocity is therefore relatively preserved. (From Bach RG, Kern MJ. Practical coronary physiology: clinical applications of the Doppler flow velocity guide wire. Cardiol Clin 1997; 15:77–99.)

Hagen-Poiseuille Law

The most fundamental law that governs the flow of fluids through cylindrical tubes was derived empirically by Poiseuille.[9] He extended the work of Bernoulli, who considered only ideal frictionless fluids, by recognizing that mechanical energy is always lost by conversion to heat in moving fluids, from one point to the next.[5,8] This energy loss is related principally to the viscosity of fluid. Poiseuille also observed, through precise measurements, that flow of fluid varies directly as the fourth power of the radius of the tube it is traveling in. As a result of his observations of the influence of the tube diameter and viscosity on the flow of liquid in pipes, he proposed the following relationship:

$$Q = \frac{\Delta P \pi r^4}{8 \eta l}$$ [equation 11]

where Q is the flow (cm^3/sec); $\Delta P = P_1 - P_2$, which represents the change in potential energy ($dynes/cm^2$) between 2 points separated by a distance of the length of the tube, 1 (cm); r is the inside radius (cm) of the tube; ηis the coefficient of viscosity expressed in dynes . sec/cm^2; andB/8 is the constant of proportionality.

This relationship can be rearranged to show that the pressure drop in a vessel is proportional to blood flow divided by the vessel radius to the fourth power[12]:

$$\Delta P = \frac{Q8\eta l}{\pi r^4} \qquad \text{[equation 12]}$$

Similar contemporary observations were made by a German hydraulic engineer, Gotthilf Hagen, whose publication actually claims priority, so that the law has now been termed the "Hagen-Poiseuille law."[8]

Although Poiseuille was interested primarily in the physical determinants of blood flow, he substituted simpler liquids for blood in his measurement of flow through glass pipes. As a result, Poiseuille's law applies only to the steady (nonpulsatile), laminar flow of Newtonian fluids through a straight cylindrical tube with rigid walls.[5,9]

Laminar Flow

When blood flows at a steady rate through a long smooth vessel, it flows in streamlines, with each layer of blood remaining the same distance from the wall. Also, the central portion of the blood stays in the center of the vessel.[13,14] Laminar flow refers to a flow pattern that may be represented as a series of infinitely thin, concentric layers or "laminae" of fluids sliding past each other, with each layer moving at a different velocity from its neighboring layers[4,9] (Fig. 2).

When laminar flow occurs, the velocity of flow in the center of the vessel is far greater than that toward the outer edges. As the fluid moves through the tube, a thin layer of fluid in contact with the tube's wall adheres to the wall and is stationary. The layer of fluid just central to this external lamina must shear against this stationary layer and moves a small distance, but with a finite velocity. Similarly, the next more central layer moves still more rapidly and for a longer distance. The longitudinal velocity profile is that of a parabaloid, and this effect is called the *parabolic profile* for the velocity of blood flow.[5,9,13]

Flow is considered fully developed when this parabolic profile exists. The velocity at the center of the stream is maximal and equal to twice the mean velocity of flow across the entire cross-section of the tube.[9] This parabolic profile can be demonstrated with a simple experiment seen in Figure 3, which shows 2 fluids in a glass pipe. If these fluids are placed in

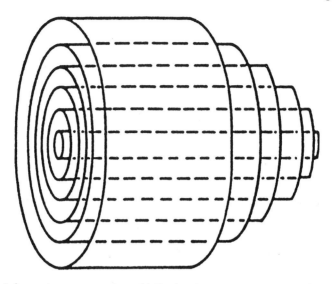

Figure 2. Schematic representation of fully developed, steady, laminar flow through a tube. Concentric layers of fluid slide on one another, with the center layers moving more rapidly than those at the periphery, resulting in a parabolic velocity profile. (From Vorp DA, Trachtenberg JD, Webster MW. Arterial hemodynamics and wall mechanics. Sem Vasc Surg 1998; 11:169–180.)

a glass pipe with no flow, their longitudinal interface is flat. However, when these same fluids flow through the glass pipe, a parabolic profile is seen to develop.

For a parabolic flow profile to develop, the tube must be long enough. When fluid passes from a large container into a smaller cylindrical tube, the velocity profile at the entrance is essentially flat (same velocity all across the tube diameter). Just beyond the entrance, friction between the stationary outermost layer and the immediately adjacent concentric layer causes the latter to slow down. This layer then slows the next layer down

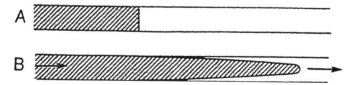

Figure 3. Experiment demonstrating parabolic blood flow with much faster flow in the center of a vessel. **A.** Two fluids before flow begins; **B.** same fluids 1 second after flow begins. (From Gayton AC, Hall JE. Textbook of Medical Physiology, 9th edition, 1996).

and so on down the tube until the "boundary layer" extends to the center of the tube. At this point, flow is considered to be fully developed and the profile is truly parabolic. The *entrance length* (L_x) in centimeters required to develop a parabolic profile is a function of the radius of the tube and the Reynolds' number (Re).

$$L_x = k \cdot r \cdot Re \qquad \text{[equation 13]}$$

where k is a constant that approximates 0.16 for Reynolds' numbers greater than 50[5]. Reynolds' number will be discussed further in this chapter with regard to turbulent flow.

Viscosity

Viscosity may be defined as the friction existing between contiguous layers of fluid. The friction is due to strong intermolecular attractions.[5] Viscosity is a major factor influencing flow. The greater the viscosity, the less the flow in a vessel if all other factors are constant.[12,13] The primary determinant of blood viscosity is the hematocrit, with viscosity increasing exponentially with increasing hematocrit. Typically the viscosity of whole blood ranges from 2 to 15 times that of water[4,13] (Fig. 4A). Other factors that increase viscosity are temperature, plasma proteins, and vessel diameter.

At body temperature, viscosity increases by roughly 2% for every 1°C drop in temperature. This is of clinical importance when hypothermia is used in surgery or is encountered as a result of cold exposure. Plasma proteins also play a role in the viscosity of blood. For example, the presence of fibrinogen enhances the flexibility of red blood cells, which in turn decreases the apparent viscosity of whole blood.[4] The viscosity of blood plasma is about 1.5 times that of water.

The diameter of the vessel may also influence blood viscosity. In vessels larger than 0.5 mm in diameter, viscosity is independent of vessel diameter; however, in the microcirculation, apparent viscosity decreases with decreasing diameter[4] (Fig. 4B). Thus, in tubes as small as the terminal arterioles, the viscosity of whole blood is as little as one half of that found in large vessels.[13] Additional factors besides hematocrit, temperature, and plasma proteins affect blood viscosity in the microcirculation.

Blood flow in minute tubes exhibits far less viscous effect than it does in large vessels. This phenomenon, known as the *Fahraeus-Lindqvist effect*, begins to appear when vessel diameter falls below about 1.5 mm. The Fahraeus-Lindqvist effect is explained by the alignment of red blood cells in the center of the flow as they move through very small vessels. This central axial accumulation results in a cell-free marginal zone along the ves-

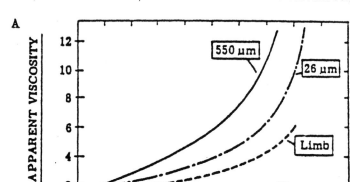

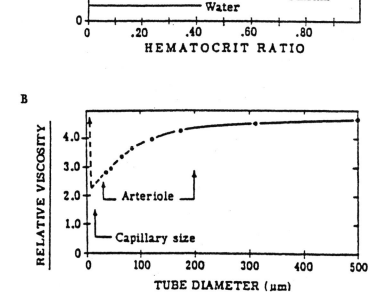

Figure 4. **A.** Variation of water, plasma, and blood viscosities with hematocrit (units in centipoise). Data for blood are given for flow through tubes of 26 μm and 550 μm, as well as through an isolated dog hind limb. **B.** Variation of blood viscosity with tube diameter. In tubes smaller than 0.5 mm (i.e., arterioles), viscosity decreases with decreasing tube diameter (the Fahraeus-Lindqvist effect). This effect is lost at the level of the capillaries. (From Vorp DA, Trachtenberg JD, Webster MW. Arterial hemodynamics and wall mechanics. Sem Vasc Surg 1988; 11:169–180.)

sel wall consisting of the less viscous plasma, as well as eliminating the viscous resistance that occurs internally in blood moving randomly. This effect is lost at the level of the capillaries because of their smaller size (4 μm diameter on average) with respect to the red blood cell (8 μm average diameter). Cells often become stuck at constrictions in small blood vessels. This happens especially in capillaries where the nuclei of endothelial cells protrude into the capillary lumen. When this occurs, blood flow can become blocked for a fraction of a second or for longer periods, giving an apparent effect of greatly increasing viscosity as increased force is required to squeeze the erythrocytes through these small vessels[4,13] (Fig. 4B). In addition, the viscosity of blood increases as its velocity decreases.[14] Because the velocity of blood flow in the small vessels is extremely slow, often less than 1 mm/sec, blood viscosity can increase as much as 10-fold from this factor alone. This effect is partly caused by adherence of the slowly moving red cells to one another (formation of rouleaux and larger aggregates), as well as to the vessel walls.[13] The converse is also true, that increased velocity reduces the viscosity, which becomes apparent in the venules where the velocity begins to increase.[12] Because some of these effects of the microcirculation decrease viscosity and others increase viscosity, it is usually assumed that the overall viscous effects in the small vessels are about equivalent to those that occur in the larger vessels.[13]

Shear Stress

For laminar flow, the force per unit area (the area parallel to the flow) tending to impede the sliding movement between layers is called *shear stress*.[4] For a given pressure difference and for a cylindrical tube of given dimensions, the flow varies as a function of the nature of fluid itself. This flow-determining property of fluids is viscosity (η), which may be interpreted as the resistance of fluid to shearing motion. Newton defined viscosity as the ratio of shear stress (τ) to the *shear rate* (D) of the fluid.[4,9,15]

$$\eta = \frac{\tau}{D} \qquad \text{[equation 14]}$$

Shear rate (D) is the ratio of the change in velocity (du) to the change in the radius (dy) between each cylindrical laminar layer.[5,16] Wall shear rate represents the ratio between the blood viscosity in the vicinity of the wall and its distance from the wall.[17]

$$D = \frac{du}{dy} \qquad \text{[equation 15]}$$

The flow of blood, by virtue of viscosity, engenders on the luminal vessel wall and endothelial surface a frictional force per unit area known as shear stress (τ).[2] Wall shear stress represents the frictional force applied by the circulating blood column on the intimal surface of vessels.[16,17]

An example of these terms given by Berne and Levy[9] may be seen in Figure 5. Consider the flow of a Newtonian fluid between 2 parallel plates. The bottom plate is stationary, and the upper plate moves along the upper

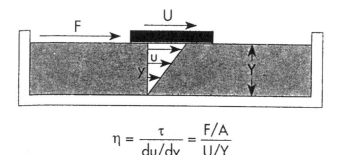

$$\eta = \frac{\tau}{du/dy} = \frac{F/A}{U/Y}$$

Figure 5. For a Newtonian fluid, the viscosity is defined as the ratio of shear stress to shear rate. For a plate of contact area, A, moving across the surface of a liquid, shear stress equals the ratio of force, F, applied in the direction of motion to the contact area, A, and shear rate equals the ratio of the velocity of the plate, U, to the depth of the liquid, Y. (From Berne RM, Levy MN. Physiology. St. Louis, Mosby, 1998.)

surface of the fluid. The shear stress, τ, is defined as the ratio of F:A, where F is the force applied to the upper plate in the direction of its motion along the upper surface of the fluid, and A is the area of the upper plate that is in contact with the fluid. The shear rate is du/dy, where u is the velocity of a minute fluid element in the direction parallel to the motion of the upper plate, and y is the distance of that fluid element above the bottom, stationary plate. For a plate that travels with a constant velocity, U, across the surface of a Newtonian fluid, the velocity profile of the fluid will be linear. The fluid layer in contact with the upper plate will adhere to it and therefore will move at the same velocity, U, as the plate. Each minute element of fluid between the plates will move at a velocity, u, that is proportional to its distance, y, from the lower plate. Therefore, the shear rate will be U/Y, where Y is the distance between the 2 plates. Because viscosity, η, is defined as the ratio of shear stress, τ, to shear rate, du/dy, in the example shown:

$$\eta = \frac{F/A}{U/Y} \qquad \text{[equation 16]}$$

The dimensions of viscosity are dynes/cm^2 divided by (cm/sec)/cm, or dynes · sec/cm^2. In honor of Poiseuille, 1 dyne . sec/cm^2 has been termed a *poise*.[9]

From the example, the force applied to the upper plate is directed parallel to the surface, exerting a shearing stress on the liquid below, and thus it produces a differential motion of each layer of liquid relative to the adjacent layers of liquid, until the flowing liquid exerts a shearing stress on the surface of the bottom plate in contact with the liquid.[9] By rearranging equation 14, shear stress equals the product of the viscosity and the shear rate.

$$\tau = \eta \cdot D \qquad \text{[equation 17]}$$

Remember that shear rate (D) is equal to the velocity of flow divided by its distance from the wall. So the greater the rate of blood flow (Q) in the vessel, the greater the shear rate near the arterial wall, and therefore the greater the shear stress (τ) that the blood exerts on the vessel wall. The shear stress acting on the vessel wall is also known as viscous drag.[9]

Poiseuille's law applies only to constant laminar flow of a Newtonian fluid in a straight rigid tube of uniform bore. However, it has been demonstrated that a poiseuillean parabolic model of velocity distribution across the arterial lumen provides a useful estimate of wall shear[16] (Fig. 6A). The magnitude of shear stress can be estimated in most of the vasculature by Poiseuille's law, which states that shear stress is proportional to the shear rate of the layers of blood near the wall and blood viscosity, and inversely proportional to the third power of the radius.[2,15,18]

$$\tau = \frac{4\eta Q}{\eta r^3}$$ [equation 18]

Measurements using different modalities show that shear stress ranges from 1 to 6 dynes/cm² in the venous system and between 10 and 70 dynes/cm² in the arterial vascular network[2] (Fig. 6B).

Although atherosclerosis is typically thought of as a systemic disease, it does not occur randomly throughout the circulatory system. In the human, atherosclerotic lesions usually predominate at the origins of tributaries, bifurcations, and curvatures. For example, highly lesion-prone areas include the coronary vascular bed, the carotid bifurcation, and the iliac arteries[3,4] (Fig. 7). In these susceptible areas, blood flow is slow and changes

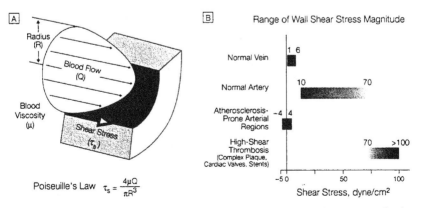

Figure 6. **A.** Cross-sectional diagram of a blood vessel showing shear stress, the frictional force per unit area acting on the inner vessel wall and on the luminal surface of the endothelium as a result of the flow of viscous blood. **B.** Tabular diagram illustrating the range of shear stress magnitude encountered in veins, arteries, and in low-shear and high-shear pathological states (From Malek AM, Alper SC, Izumo S. Hemodynamic shear stress and its role in atherosclerosis. JAMA 1999; 282:2035–2042.)

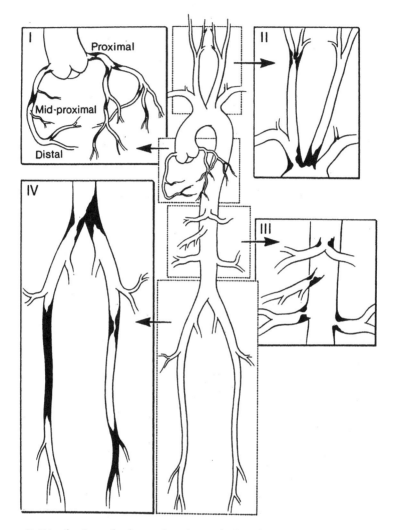

Figure 7. Distribution of atherosclerotic occlusive disease. (From DeBakey ME, Lawrie GM, Glaeser DH. Patterns of atherosclerosis and their surgical significance. Ann Surg 1985; 201:115–131.)

direction with the cardiac cycle, resulting in a weak net hemodynamic shear stress. Thus, the preferred sites for the formation of atherosclerotic plaques and wall thickening are located in regions of slow flow and low wall shear stress.[1,14] In contrast, vessel regions that are exposed to steady blood flow and a higher magnitude of shear stress remain relatively disease free.[2]

Shear stress has also been shown to actively influence vessel wall re-modeling.[1,2,4,16–19] Specifically, chronic increases in blood flow, and consequently shear stress, lead to the expansion of the luminal radius such that mean shear stress is returned to its baseline level. Conversely, decreased shear stress resulting from lower flow or blood viscosity induces a decrease in internal vessel radius. The net effect of these endothelial-mediated compensatory responses is the maintenance of mean arterial hemodynamic shear stress magnitude at approximately 15 to 20 dynes/cm^2.[2]

Turbulent Flow

In laminar flow, fluid elements remain in distinct laminae. However, when the rate of blood flow becomes too great, when it passes an obstruction in a vessel, when it makes a sharp turn, or when it passes over a rough surface, turbulent flow may develop. Under such conditions, fluid elements do not remain confined to definite laminae, but rapid radial mixing occurs. Turbulent flow is defined as the random motion of fluid particles.[4,13] This results in the generation of swirls in the blood, called eddy currents, and a loss of kinetic (driving) energy of the flow as the blood flows crosswise in the vessel as well as along the vessel. Therefore, for a given pressure gradient, less bulk flow is achieved under turbulent conditions, and a considerably greater pressure is required to force a given flow of fluid through the same tube when the flow is turbulent than when it is laminar. In turbulent flow, the pressure drop is approximately proportional to the square of the flow rate, whereas in laminar flow the pressure drop is proportional to the first power of the flow rate. Hence, to produce a given flow, a pump such as the heart must do considerably more work if turbulence develops.

Flow is predominantly laminar in a healthy circulatory system, with the exception of small bursts of turbulence in the aorta. However, the normally laminar flow may become transitional or turbulent in the presence of stenosis. Also, the effect of even a small amount of turbulence may play a very important role in the pathophysiology of thrombus formation and vascular disease.[20] Turbulent flow may be associated with stagnation points on the vascular wall and can also cause excessively high or low wall shear stresses compared with laminar flow.[4]

The point at which flow changes from laminar to turbulent is estimated by using the *Reynolds' number* (Re), a dimensionless parameter, which is calculated from the mean flow velocity multiplied by the diameter of the vessel and divided by the kinematic viscosity.

$$Re = \frac{vd}{v} \qquad \text{[equation 19]}$$

The kinematic viscosity (v) is equal to the viscosity of the fluid divided by the density of the fluid ($v = \eta/\rho$). Reynolds' number physically represents the ratio of inertial forces acting on a fluid to the viscous forces. The numerator represents the inertial forces and the denominator represents the viscous forces. The numerator will be large when flow is rapid and small when flow is slow. The higher the Reynolds' number, the more likely it is for the flow to be turbulent, because inertial forces increase and predominate over viscous forces.[21]

When Reynolds' number rises above 200 to 400, turbulent flow occurs at some branches of vessels, but dies out along the smooth portions of the vessel after the entrance length (L_x) is met. When Reynolds' number rises above 2000, turbulence usually occurs, even in a straight smooth vessel.[13] Reynolds demonstrated that in straight tubes with steady flow and Reynolds' numbers less than 2000, laminar flow was stable. For Reynolds' numbers greater than 2000 laminar flow was possible; however, once disturbed, the flow would become turbulent with the associated dramatic increase in pressure gradient, and this turbulence would persist. Thus, below a critical pressure gradient, the flow rate is proportional to the driving pressure gradient (Poiseuille's law). Above the critical pressure gradient, the flow rate may increase, but if it is disturbed, it will not increase in a predictable way until the pressure gradient exceeds a turbulence threshold (Fig. 8). Experiments using blood flowing through rigid tubes found the critical Reynolds' number to be approximately 2000, showing that blood in this respect has properties of a homogeneous fluid.[21]

The equation for Reynolds' number illustrates the potential physical and clinical factors responsible for the generation of turbulent flow: smaller vessel diameter (d), seen in regions of stenosis; lower fluid viscosity (η), seen in anemia; and increased flow (Q), seen with exertion. In addition to these factors, turbulence may be caused by sudden changes in vessel size or geometry, such as at bifurcations or anastamoses, or by irregularities in the vessel wall created by atherosclerotic plaque.[4]

In addition to laminar and turbulent flow, recent evidence suggests that spiral or helical-type flow patterns may exist.[22–24] This laminar vortical flow may even exist in different directions, with the blood rotation being counterclockwise or clockwise in different parts of the circulation.[22] Further work with this type of blood flow is required, although the spiral pattern of disease seen in the left anterior descending and left circumflex coronary arteries[23] has led some to believe it exists. However, discussion of spiral blood flow is beyond the scope of this chapter.

Resistance

Resistance is defined as the impediment to blood flow in a vessel, but it cannot be measured by direct means. Instead, resistance must be calcu-

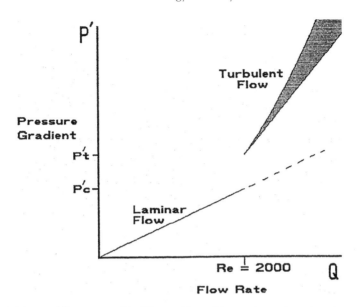

Figure 8. Types of flow seen with different Reynolds numbers plotted against various pressure gradients. The laminar flow curve is representative of Poiseuille's law, where below a critical pressure (P'c) the flow rate is proportional to the driving pressure gradient. The shape of turbulent flow depends on tube radius, roughness of the wall, fluid density, and viscosity, and does not increase in a predictable way until the pressure gradient exceeds the turbulence threshold (P't). (From Papanicolaou G, Beach KW, Zierle RE, Strandness DE. Systolic flow limitation in stenotic lower-extremity vein-grafts. J Vasc Surg 1996; 23:394–400.)

lated from measurements of blood flow and pressure differences in the vessel.[13] The hemodynamic behavior of each resistance element in the circulation can be described by using an analogy of *Ohm's law* from electrical theory. Ohm's law states that resistance in a circuit is equal to the voltage drop, E_1-E_2, across an element divided by the current flow, I.[9,25]

$$R = \frac{E_1 - E_2}{I}$$ [equation 20]

For fluid mechanics, the hydraulic resistance, R, may be defined as the ratio of pressure drop, P_1-P_2, to flow, Q.[9,26]

$$R = \frac{P_1 - P_2}{Q}$$ [equation 21]

However, unlike electrical resistance, hemodynamic resistance does not remain constant over a wide range of flows. In theory, the minimal possible resistance of a vessel can be estimated from its length and radius by applying Poiseuille's law.[5,9,11]

$$R_{min} = \frac{8\eta l}{\pi r^4}$$
[equation 22]

Because resistance varies inversely as the fourth power of the radius of the vessel, the principle determinant of the resistance to blood flow through any individual vessel within the circulatory system is the caliber of the vessel. At low flows, resistance is constant and is given by Poiseuille's law. However, because of additional energy losses related to acceleration, disturbed flow, and turbulence, the resistance of a given vascular segment tends to increase as flow velocity increases, provided that there is no concomitant change in vascular diameter.[5,9,25]

Resistance within the circulatory system is encountered either in series or in parallel. For resistances in series, the total resistance, R_t, of the entire system equals the sum of the individual resistances.

$$R_t = R_1 + R_2 + \ldots + Rn$$
[equation 23]

For resistances in series, the pressure drop across the entire system, or the difference between inflow pressure, P_i, and outflow pressure, P_o, is equal to the sum of the pressure drops across each of the individual resistances. Under steady-state conditions, the flow, Q, through any given cross-section must equal the flow through any other cross-section.[9] By dividing the pressure drop over each resistance in series by the flow, and adding each individual resistance, the total resistance of the system is derived. This is illustrated in the system shown in Figure 9.

For resistances in parallel, the inflow and outflow pressures are the same for the entire system. Under steady-state conditions, the total flow,

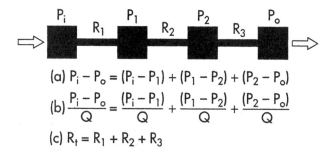

(a) $P_i - P_o = (P_i - P_1) + (P_1 - P_2) + (P_2 - P_o)$

(b) $\dfrac{P_i - P_o}{Q} = \dfrac{(P_i - P_1)}{Q} + \dfrac{(P_1 - P_2)}{Q} + \dfrac{(P_2 - P_o)}{Q}$

(c) $R_t = R_1 + R_2 + R_3$

Figure 9. For resistances arranged in series, the total resistance equals the sum of the individual resistances. P_i = inflow pressure; P_o = outflow pressure; Q = flow. (From Berne RM, Levy MN. Physiology. St. Louis, Mosby, 1998.)

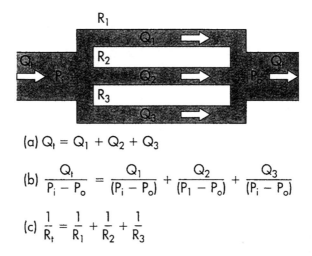

(a) $Q_t = Q_1 + Q_2 + Q_3$

(b) $\dfrac{Q_t}{P_i - P_o} = \dfrac{Q_1}{(P_i - P_o)} + \dfrac{Q_2}{(P_1 - P_o)} + \dfrac{Q_3}{(P_i - P_o)}$

(c) $\dfrac{1}{R_t} = \dfrac{1}{R_1} + \dfrac{1}{R_2} + \dfrac{1}{R_3}$

Figure 10. For resistances arranged in parallel, the reciprocal of the total resistance equals the sum of the reciprocals of the individual resistances. P_i = inflow pressure; P_o = outflow pressure; Q = flow. (From Berne RM, Levy MN. Physiology. St. Louis, Mosby, 1998.)

Q_t, through the system equals the sum of the flows through the individual parallel elements. Because the pressure gradient is the same for all parallel elements, the different flows may be divided by the pressure gradient to give the reciprocal of total resistance (Fig. 10). For resistances in parallel, the reciprocal of the total resistance equals the sum of the reciprocals of the individual resistances.[9]

$$\frac{1}{R_t} = \frac{1}{R_1} + \frac{1}{R_2} + \dots + \frac{1}{R_n} \qquad \text{[equation 24]}$$

The term *conductance* is another way of stating this relationship. Conductance is a measure of the blood flow through a vessel for a given pressure difference, and is equal to the reciprocal of the resistance.

$$\text{Conductance} = \frac{1}{\text{resistance}} \qquad \text{[equation 25]}$$

Thus, for vessels in parallel, the total conductance is the sum of the individual conductances.[9,13]

The dimensions of hemodynamic resistance are dynes . $\sec/cm^5$. It is usually more convenient, however, to use the peripheral resistance unit (PRU), which is mm $Hg/mL/sec^5$. So, if the pressure difference between 2 points in a vessel is 1 mm Hg and the flow is 1 mL/sec, the resistance is said to be 1 PRU. The total peripheral resistance in the human body is also approximately 1 PRU. The rate of blood flow through the circulation when a person is at rest is close to 100 mL/sec, and the pressure difference from the systemic arteries to the systemic veins is about 100 mm Hg. Therefore, the resistance of the entire circulatory system is about 100 mm Hg/100 mL/sec or 1 PRU.

Viscoelasticity

The components of the circulatory system are not rigid tubes, but distensible vessels. The distensible nature of the arteries allows them to accommodate the pulsatile output of the heart and to average out the pressure pulsations. This provides an almost completely smooth, continuous flow of blood through the very small blood vessels of the tissues.[7] Because the heart pumps intermittently, the entire stroke volume is discharged into the arterial system during systole. Systole usually occupies only about one third of the cardiac cycle. In fact, most of the stroke volume is actually pumped during the rapid ejection phase, which constitutes about half of systole. A small part of the energy of cardiac contraction is dissipated as forward capillary flow during systole. The remainder is stored as potential energy, as much of the stroke volume is retained by the distensible arteries. During diastole, the elastic recoil of the arterial walls converts this potential energy into capillary blood flow. Thus, continuous perfusion of organs and tissues is ensured. If the arterial walls were rigid, capillary flow would not occur during diastole.[27,28]

This dampening effect is related to the viscoelastic properties of arterial walls. It is termed the *Windkessel model* of the circulation,[27-29] named after the Windkessels of antique fire engines. The Windkessels contained a large volume of trapped air. The compressibility of the air that remained trapped above the water in the Windkessel converted the intermittent inflow of water from the water source to a steady outflow of water at the nozzle of the fire hose.[27] The same is seen in the circulation where the intermittent stroke volume from the heart in systole is converted to a steady capillary blood flow throughout the cardiac cycle.

Vascular distensibility is normally expressed as the fractional increase in volume (ΔV) for each millimeter of mercury rise in pressure (ΔP).

$$\text{vascular distensibility} = \frac{\text{increase in volume}}{\text{increase in pressure x original volume}}$$

$$= \frac{\Delta V}{\Delta P \cdot V} \qquad \text{[equation 26]}$$

where V equals the original volume. Thus, if 1 mm Hg caused a vessel that originally contained 10 mL of blood to increase its volume by 1 mL, the distensibility would equal 0.1 per mm Hg, or 10% per mm Hg.[7]

In hemodynamic studies, it is usually much more important to know the total quantity of blood that can be stored in a given portion of the circulation for each millimeter of mercury pressure rise than to know the distensibility of the individual vessels.[7] This value is termed *compliance* (C), which is defined as the increase in volume (ΔV) divided by the increase in pressure (ΔP).

$$C = \frac{\Delta V}{\Delta P}$$ [equation 27]

Vascular compliance is often reported using fractional changes in area or diameter instead of volume because these quantities are easier to measure.[4]

Compliance and distensibility are quite different. A highly distensible vessel that has a slight volume may have far less compliance than a much less distensible vessel that has a large volume because compliance is equal to distensibility times volume.[7]

Compliance is an intrinsic property of the vascular wall, dependent on the material stiffness, vascular tone, matrix content, and calcifications.[4] *Young's modulus of elasticity* (E_p) is a measure of the stiffness of an elastic material. It is equal to the ratio of applied stress (τ) to the resulting strain (ε).

$$E_p = \frac{\tau}{\varepsilon}$$ [equation 28]

The circumferential stress applied to an arterial wall is a function of the transmural pressure (intraluminal pressure minus the extravascular pressure), the inside radius of the artery, r_i, and its wall thickness, δ.

$$\tau = \frac{\Delta P \cdot r_i}{\delta}$$ [equation 29]

where pressure is in dynes/cm^2, and r_i and Δ are in centimeters. Circumferential strain, e, is proportional to the ratio of the change in outside radius, δr_o, to the original outside radius, r_o.

$$\varepsilon = \frac{\Delta r_o}{r_o}$$ [equation 30]

The equations for circumferential stress (equation 29) and circumferential strain (equation 30) are substituted into the equation for the elastic modules (equation 28) to yield:

$$Ep = \frac{\Delta P \cdot r_o \cdot r_i}{\Delta r_o \delta} \qquad \text{[equation 31]}$$

Although wall thickness is an important determinant of the changes in volume or radius of the vessel wall for a given change in pressure, it is difficult to obtain accurate measurements of arterial wall thickness. For this reason, Young's elastic modulus can be approximated[5,7] by:

$$Ep = \frac{\Delta P r_o}{\Delta r_o} \qquad \text{[equation 32]}$$

By using the fractional changes in diameter $(r_o/\Delta r_o)$ of a vessel to estimate the change in volume (ΔV) of the vessel, Young's modulus of elasticity can be seen to be the reciprocal of compliance:

$$Ep = \frac{\Delta P}{\Delta V} \qquad \text{[equation 33]}$$

Given the above description of compliance as the reciprocal of the elastic modulus, it becomes apparent that for vessels of identical inner diameter and composition, the thicker vessel will be less compliant due to the effect of wall thickness (δ) on the circumferential stress. Other factors that have been shown to decrease compliance of the arteries are the pressure range at which arteries are subjected,[4,5,17,30,31] aging,[4,5,27] cardiovascular risk factors such as hypertension and hypercholesterolemia,[14] and the effects of vasoactive substances.[17,28]

Compliance is dependent on the pressure range over which it is measured. Arteries are most compliant under diastolic pressure, then they gradually stiffen (become less compliant) as pressure increases. Two fibrous proteins, elastin and collagen, determine the mechanical properties of the arterial wall. The highly elastic elastin fibers in the arterial wall are responsible for the high compliance of an artery at low transmural pressures (<50 to 75 mm Hg), while at higher pressures, the stiffer collagen fibers are gradually drawn taught and the compliance decreases logarithmically as the effective rigidity increases.[4,5,17,28] This diminished compliance at high pressures is caused by the fact that collagen fibers aligned around the arterial circumference are tortuous at low pressures and are gradually stretched out during distension, causing a reinforcement and stiffening of the wall at high pressures.[4] Therefore, the typical pressure-volume curve of arteries has 2 phases: (1) a low-pressure, compliant part, and (2) a high-pressure, stiff part (Fig. 11). The compliance at any point on the curve is represented by the slope, $\Delta V / \Delta P$, at that point, and the elastic modulus is represented by the slope, $\Delta P / \Delta V$. The increasing elastic modulus and the decreasing compliance with aging both reflect the stiffness of the arterial walls as individuals age. Compliance depends partly on blood pressure, but more importantly on the intrinsic elastic properties and composition of the arterial wall.

Atherosclerosis remains the leading cause of death in the developed world. Hemodynamic factors have been shown to be associated with the genesis, progression, and regression of atherosclerotic plaques both in native vessels and in bypass grafts. To fully understand how atherosclerosis affects the vascular system, the clinician must have a fundamental knowledge of the rheological principles and equations that pertain to normal blood flow and how it is altered in various pathological states.

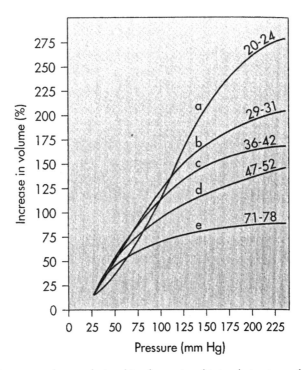

Figure 11. Pressure-volume relationships for aortas obtained at autopsy from humans in different age groups (denoted by the numbers at the right of each of the curves). (From Berne RM, Levy MN. Physiology. St. Louis, Mosby, 1998.)

References

1. Asakura T, Karino T. Flow patterns and spatial distribution of atherosclerotic lesions in human coronary arteries. Circ Res 1990; 66:1045–1066.
2. Malek AM, Alper SL, Izumo S. Hemodynamic shear stress and its role in atherosclerosis. JAMA 1999; 282:2035–2042.
3. Thubrikar MJ, Robiscsek F. Pressure-induced arterial wall stress and atherosclerosis. Ann Thorac Surg 1995; 59:1594–1603.
4. Vorp DA, Trachtenberg JD, Webster MW. Arterial hemodynamics and wall mechanics. Sem Vasc Surg 1998; 11:169–180.
5. Sumner DS. Essential hemodynamic principles. In Rutherford RB (ed): Vascular Surgery, 15th ed. Philadelphia, W.B. Saunders, 2000.
6. Milnor WR. Pulsatile blood flow. N Engl J Med 1972; 287:27–34.
7. Guyton AC, Hall JE. Vascular distensibility, and functions of the arterial and venous systems. In Guyton AC, Hall JE: Textbook of Medical Physiology, 9th ed. Philadelphia, W.B. Saunders, 1996.
8. Hopkins RW. Presidential address: Energy, Poise, and Resilience: Daniel Bernoulli, Thomas Young, J.L.M. Poiseuille, and F.A. Simone. J Vasc Surg 1991; 13:777–784.
9. Berne RM, Levy MN. Hemodynamics. In Berne RM, Levy MN: Physiology. St. Louis, Mosby, 1998.
10. Bach RG, Kern MJ. Practical coronary physiology: clinical application of the Doppler flow velocity guide wire. Cardiol Clin 1997; 15:77–99.
11. Ofili EO, Kern MJ, Vrain JA, Donohue TJ, Bach R, et al. Differential characterization of blood flow, velocity, and vascular resistance between proximal and distal normal epicardial human coronary arteries: analysis by intracoronary Doppler spectral flow velocity. Am J Heart 1995; 130:37–46.
12. Groebe K. Precapillary servo control of blood pressure and postcapillary adjustment of flow to tissue metabolic stress. Circulation 1996; 94:1876–1885.
13. Guyton AC, Hall JE. Overview of the circulation: medical physics of pressure, flow, and resistance. In Guyton AC, Hall JE: Textbook of Medical Physiology, 9th ed. Philadelphia, W.B. Saunders, 1996.
14. Sabbah HN, Khaja F, Brymer JF, Hawkins ET, Stein PD. Blood velocity in the right coronary artery: relation to the distribution of atherosclerotic lesions. Am J Cardiol 1984; 53:1008–1012.
15. Hoeks APG, Samijo SK, Brands PJ, Reneman RS. Noninvasive determination of shear-rate distribution across the arterial lumen. Hypertension 1995; 26:26–33.
16. Gnasso A, Carallo C, Irace C, Spagnuolo V, De Novara G, et al. Association between intima-media thickness and wall shear stress in common carotid arteries in healthy male subjects. Circulation 1996; 94:3257–3262.
17. Levenson J, Pithois-Merli I, Simon A. Mechanical factors in large artery disease and antihypertensive drugs. Am J Cardiol 1990; 66:39C–42C.
18. Sterpetti AV, Cucina A, D'Angelo LS, Cardillo B, Cavallaro A. Shear stress modulates the proliferation rate, protein synthesis, and mitogenic activity of arterial smooth muscle cells. Surgery 1993; 113:691–699.
19. Nwasokwa ON, Weiss M, Gladstone C, Bodenheimer MM. Effect of coronary artery size on the prevalence of atherosclerosis. Am J Cardiol 1996; 78:741–746.
20. Wong PKC, Eng B, Johnston KW, Ethier CR, Cobbold RSC. Computer simulation of blood flow patterns in arteries of various geometries. J Vasc Surg 1991; 14:658–667.

21. Papanicolaou G, Beach KW, Zierler RE, Strandness DE. Systolic flow limitation in stenotic lower-extremity vein grafts. J Vasc Surg 1996; 23:394–400.
22. Zakharov VN. Structural analysis of moving blood from the viewpoint of new principles of circulation mechanics. J Cardiovasc Surg 1994; 35:19–26.
23. Bargeron CB, Deters OJ, Mark FF, Friedman MH. Effect of flow partition on wall shear in a cast of a human coronary artery. Cardiovasc Res 1988; 22:340–344.
24. He X, Ku DN. Pulsatile flow in the human left coronary artery bifurcation: average conditions. J Biomech Eng 1996; 118:74–82.
25. Tyberg JV, Massie BM, Botvinick EH. The hemodynamics of coronary arterial stenosis. Cardivasc Clin 1977; 8:71–84.
26. Louagie YAG, Haxhe JP, Jamart J, Buche M, Schoevaerdts JC. Intraoperative assessment of coronary artery bypass grafts using a pulsed Doppler flowmeter. Ann Thorac Surg 1994; 58:742–749.
27. Berne RM, Levy MN. The arterial system. In Berne RM, Levy MN: Physiology. St. Louis, Mosby, 1998.
28. Marchais SJ, Guerin AP, Pannier B, Delavaud G, London GM. Arterial compliance and blood pressure. Drugs 1993; 46(suppl 2):82–87.
29. Cohn JN, Finkelstein SM. Abnormalities of vascular compliance in hypertension, aging, and heart failure. J Hyperten 1992; 10(suppl 6):S61–S64.
30. Dzau VJ, Safar ME. Large conduit arteries in hypertension: role of the vascular renin-angiotensin system. Circulation 1988; 77:947–954.
31. DeBakey ME, Lawrie GM, Glaeser DH. Patterns of atherosclerosis and their surgical significance. Ann Surg 1985; 201:115–131.

2

Functional and Anatomical Tests to Evaluate Graft Patency after Vascular Surgery Procedures:

Principles and Clinical Applications

Einar Stranden, PhD

Introduction

The need to measure blood flow intraoperatively became apparent during the development of reconstructive arterial surgery. However, many surgeons unfortunately still rely on pulse palpation as an index of flow, not realizing that a vessel can pulsate even when there is no blood flowing through it. In fact, if the vessel occludes distal to the palpation site, the pulse may even increase, though admittedly not for long (Fig. 1).

The primary aim in flowmetry is to obtain information on the immediate result of the reconstruction, where a technical failure may jeopardize an otherwise successful operation. There is a clear correlation between the blood flow values obtained following injection of papaverine and the prognosis of the arterial reconstruction. Dedichen[1] found that the risk of early postoperative occlusion was significantly increased if the basal blood flow after reconstruction was less than 100 mL/min or the papaverine-induced flow was less than 200 mL/min. However, it can be ques-

From: D'Ancona G, Karamanoukian HL, Ricci M, Salerno TA, Bergsland J (eds). *Intraoperative Graft Patency Verification in Cardiac and Vascular Surgery.* © Futura Publishing Company, Armonk, NY, 2001.

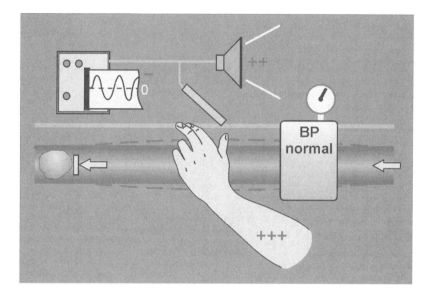

Figure 1. Pulse palpation is a poor indicator of blood flow. If the artery is occluded distal to the palpation, the pulse is increased compared to an open artery. Because the artery is compliant, there is some blood flow back and forth into the occluded segment. This movement might produce a Doppler sound interpreted as normal, whereas the spectrum more correctly shows a reverberant flow with zero mean blood flow.

tioned whether the flow measurements are sensitive enough to detect minor technical failures since normal blood flow values have been measured despite extensive defects at the anastomosis.[2] Furthermore, the levels of blood flow recorded during an operation may have little relation to normal activity. Under some types of anesthesia and conditions due to acute blood loss, blood flow is likely to be markedly depressed, whereas hyperemia is observed in others (epidural anesthesia).

The *basal* blood flow after bypass grafting is of limited help to precisely evaluate the arterial reconstruction, since it depends on various factors in addition to the graft itself, like arteriolar tone, blood volume, body temperature, type of anesthesia, etc. The blood flow increase observed following administration of a vasodilating agent such as papaverine or iloprost[3–5] is a significantly better indicator of the long-term prognosis, and is better suited for the detection of technical failures.

Five-year patency of femorodistal bypasses varies between 40% and 70% in many series. Some of the reocclusions may be due to intimal hyperplasia, whereas others are caused by technical failures leading to secondary thrombosis formation and graft occlusion. To eliminate technical failures, intraoperative control of the reconstruction is important. Furthermore, such investigations can also be helpful in planning the procedure and in giving an indication of the long-term prognosis of the operation.

In cardiac surgery, flowmetry was introduced at an early stage to indicate severity of disease, and to assess patency of coronary bypass grafting and the prognosis of therapy.[6–12] In coronary surgery, flowmetry is still regarded an essential tool for evaluating the anastomotic sites,[13,14] and guidelines for performing and interpreting flowmetry procedures have been developed.[15]

The purpose of this presentation is to review methods for evaluation of arterial reconstructions, and to discuss which methods are going to be important in the future.

Functional Tests

Electromagnetic Flowmeter

Electromagnetic flowmetry quantitates blood flow in a single vessel. The technique is based on the principles of electromagnetic induction, described by William Faraday 170 years ago. If an electrolyte (such as blood) flows at right angles to a magnetic field, then an electromotive force is induced in a plane, which is mutually perpendicular to the magnetic field and to the direction of fluid flow (Fig. 2). Two electrodes situated in the appropriate plane and connected to a suitable detector circuit can measure the induced voltage, which is proportional to the strength of the magnetic field and to the velocity of blood flow within the blood vessel. For most clinical and experimental applications, the probe is C-shaped so it can be slipped around the vessel. The probe must be carefully chosen so it fits tightly around the vessel to ensure a good contact between the electrodes and the vessel wall, but so that it does not compress it. The probe is designed to produce an even magnetic field, ensuring accurate measurements. Incorporated in most electromagnetic flowmeter transducers is the electromagnet in addition to the 2 recording electrodes (Fig. 3B). As the probes are manufactured for specific vessel diameters, a set of different sized probes is needed. Most flowmeters utilize an alternating magnetic field to avoid polarization of the detector electrodes.[16]

One important factor is zero stability. When recording from peripheral vessels, occluding the vessel with a clamp can check the zero reading. However, this is often impossible when flowmeters are used on the aorta or pulmonary artery.

Apart from the establishment of a true baseline, the most important criteria for accurate flow measurement are adequate linearity calibrations.[17] Ideally, and especially when applied to atheromatous vessels, each

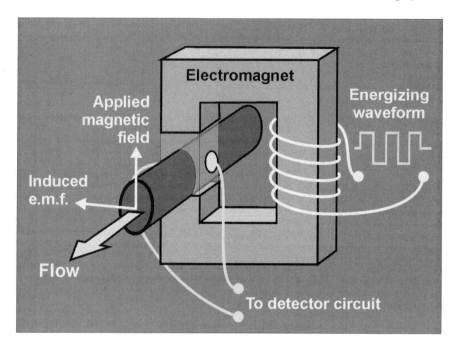

Figure 2. The principle of electromagnetic flowmetry. e.m.f. = electromotive force.

probe should be calibrated at the time and at the site of measurement. Most flowmeters are not ideally suited for doing this (Sykes, 1971), whereas with the Nycotron flowmeter (Fig. 3A) (as used by Cappelen,[6,7,9] Hall,[11] Cronestrand,[8] and Dedichen[1,3]) this procedure is relatively simple to execute in the operating theater, by using an integrator built into the instrument.

Ideally, the profile of the flow being measured should possess rotational symmetry. A concentration of flow near the electrodes causes a large increase in sensitivity, while flow concentration along the sidewalls, 90° to the electrodes, creates a decrease. One way of reducing this problem is to make the electrodes larger, covering a larger portion of the circumference. No one has thus far used such an approach. A practical adaptation is to attach the probe on a section of the vessel with assumed laminar flow, i.e., at a relatively straight-line portion of the vessel, at a distance from side branches or flow dividers.

Another source of error in making electromagnetic flow measurements is the variation in sensitivity that is observed with changing hematocrit,[18,19] influencing several commercial flowmeters. Consequently, whenever possible, the instrument should be calibrated for the particular patient. The sensitivity to hematocrit is largely due to the changing electrical impedance of blood, which also changes when blood is moved from a state of rest, as the erythrocytes tend to move to the center of the vessel (axial accumulation). This supposedly leaves a plasma layer at the vessel wall.

Recording of blood flow in expanded PTFE grafts with electromagnetic flowmetry is limited by the electrical isolation of the graft material.[20] In patients with such graft material, measurements are usually performed in the native vessel proximal to the proximal anastomosis or distal to the distal anastomosis.

Flow probes are relatively robust and have been implanted for long-term experiments in animals. However, regular inspections of their performance are desirable. It is important that the 2 electrodes be carefully cleaned and gently polished if measurements are unstable.

Ultrasound Techniques

Sound waves are pulsating pressure waves, and when above audible, e.g., above 20,000 Hz, they are termed *ultrasound*. They propagate through various media by a cyclical alteration between higher and lower particle densities. The sound is characterized by:

- Intensity, i.e., sound pressure or pressure amplitude.
- Frequency, i.e., number of oscillations per second (Hz). Audible sound is between 20 and 20,000 Hz. Medical ultrasound normally ranges be-

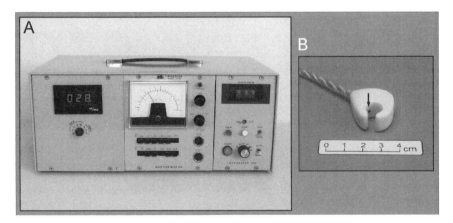

Figure 3. The Nycotron electromagnetic flowmeter (**A**) (Nycotron, Drammen, Norway) with the flow unit in the middle, and the integrator used for calibration to the right. **B**. The electromagnetic flow probe for 8-mm vessels. The arrow points at 1 of the 2 surface electrodes.

tween 2 and 10 MHz (mega Hz = million Hz), although intravascular ultrasound (IVUS) equipment may use ultrasound frequencies of 30 MHz.

- Wavelength (λ), i.e., distance between 2 adjacent maximal or minimal sound pressure levels.

An important property of the medium where the sound propagates is the specific ultrasound velocity (c). In air, this is approximately 340 m/sec, in water it is approximately 1500 m/sec. Human tissue is similar to water and the sound velocity is approximately 1540 m/sec. The wavelength is the ratio between velocity and frequency (f): $\lambda = c/f$. For medical ultrasound in human tissue λ is 0.15–0.75 mm (for audible sound λ is between 2 cm and 20 m), dependent on the frequency used.

Ultrasound energy is generated by the use of piezoelectric ceramics with electric wires on each side (transducer). The ceramic is compressed and expanded in parallel with an applied oscillating voltage, acting like a loudspeaker. On the other hand, if the ceramic is compressed and expanded by a sound wave, a variation in voltage is generated, and the ceramic acts as a microphone.

Resolution

Resolution is the ability to detect details. In an ultrasound system, there is a clear distinction between axial (along the sound wave) and lateral resolution (90° to the sound wave). Axial resolution is usually higher than lateral. It is dependent on the frequency of the emitted ultrasound (the higher the frequency, the more detailed the image), but independent of the depth of the measurement. Lateral resolution is dependent on wavelength and probe size, and decreases (lateral point size increases) with increasing depth (Fig. 4). Consequently, the ultrasound image is sharpest in the focus area of the transducer and gets more blurred in greater depths.[21]

Signal Attenuation

The signal *intensity* depends on the attenuation of the ultrasound energy as it passes through the tissue. The attenuation is dependent on *reflection, scattering*, and *absorption*.

Reflection

A sound wave hitting a medium with different acoustic impedance (the ease of which the sound wave travels within the medium) than soft

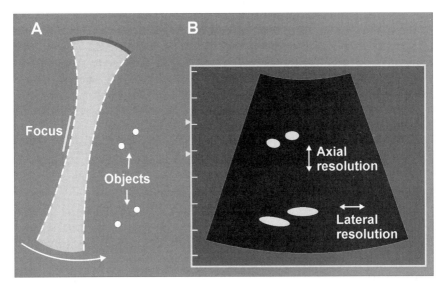

Figure 4. Spatial resolution in ultrasound consists of axial and lateral resolutions. The imaging of point targets results in a smeared image. Note that the lateral resolution is poorer than axial resolution, and that it is dependent on depth, unlike axial resolution. (Redrawn from Angelsen.[21])

tissue may be reflected. The greater the difference in impedance, the stronger is the reflection. This occurs in the boundary layers between tissue and, respectively, bone and air, for instance, against bowel gas. Ultrasound gel is used to eliminate the layer of air between the transducer and skin surface, thereby avoiding reflection of the ultrasound. However, reflection per se is not always undesirable. In fact, a reflection from boundaries within the tissue is the very basis for generating images with anatomical information in B-mode scanners.

Scattering

When a reflecting object is small compared to the wavelength, a portion of the wave energy is scattered in all directions. As scattering is proportional to the 4th power of the frequency, the attenuation increases steeply with increasing frequency.

Absorption

As the sound wave travels through tissue some of the energy is converted to heat by absorption. Absorption is proportional to the 1st power of the frequency.

The selection of a specific frequency for various diagnostic procedures always involves a compromise between the optimal ultrasound penetration depth (lower frequency–higher penetration depth), and the ability to identify relevant tissue changes (higher frequency–better sharpness or resolution). For cardiology and abdominal examinations, transducers with frequencies between 2.5 and 3.5 MHz are chosen. For obstetrics 3.5–5.0 MHz, and for peripheral vessel examinations 5.0–10.0 MHz probes are normally preferred.

The Doppler Principle

When an object moves relative to a sound source transmitting a given frequency (e.g., an ultrasound transducer), the frequency of the backscattered ultrasound is different from the emitted sound. There is a higher frequency if the movement is toward the transducer, and a lower frequency if the movement is away from the transducer (Fig. 5). This change in frequency is called Doppler shift ($\triangle f$) and is described by the equation:

$$\Delta f = 2\, f_e \cdot v \cdot \cos \theta / c \qquad \text{[equation 1]}$$

where f_e is the emitted frequency, v is the velocity of the moving objects (usually red blood cells in circulating blood) θ is the angle between the ultrasound beam and the vascular axis, and c is the speed of sound in the tissue (approximately 1540 m/sec). When using a pencil-probe Doppler transducer, θ is usually not known and may represent an error in recording blood velocity. In duplex scanners, however, θ is compensated by visual angle correction, and the velocity calculation is thus more accurate.

Small "pocket Doppler" units are usually continuous wave (CW) Doppler velocity detectors. These include 2 piezoelectric elements with overlapping ultrasound fields: one that *continuously* emits ultrasound, whereas the other is *continuously* detecting sound waves (Fig. 6). The overlap field represents the area where Doppler signals may be detected, and is termed *sample volume*. CW Doppler has no range resolution and cannot distinguish among signals from different vessels lying along the path of the beam.

Pulsed wave (PW) Doppler systems are used to detect blood velocities at specific depths. Using only 1 piezoelectric element, the transducer functions alternatingly as transducer and receiver. The received signal is sampled at an adjustable delay after pulse transmission. In this way, signals at a given depth in tissue are selected (sample volume, Fig. 6). The sample volume size is variable and is determined both by the characteristics of the ultrasound beam and by the duration of the ultrasound pulse.

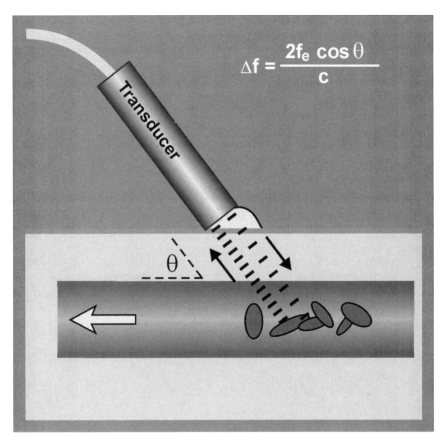

$$\Delta f = \frac{2f_e \cos \theta}{c}$$

Figure 5. Schematic drawing of a Doppler velocity detector. An ultrasound beam is transmitted by the transducer. Echoes from particles that have a movement relative to the transducer contain frequencies different from the transmitted frequency. The change in frequency, the Doppler shift (Δf), is given by the formula, where f_e is the emitted frequency, v is the velocity of the scatters, 2 is the angle between the ultrasound beam and the velocity vectors in the vessel, and c is the speed of sound in the tissue.

Shorter pulse length (shorter "packets") during the transmission phase results in a smaller sample volume, with a corresponding increase in the axial resolution.[22]

The pulsing of the beam, however, may introduce a problem when measuring large blood velocities, termed *frequency aliasing*. To avoid aliasing, the Doppler shift must be less than half the pulse repetition frequency (PRF), often referred to as the Nyquist limit of the frequency. A new transmission pulse is not allowed until the former pulse is sampled. At larger sampling depths, the time between transmission and gating has to be

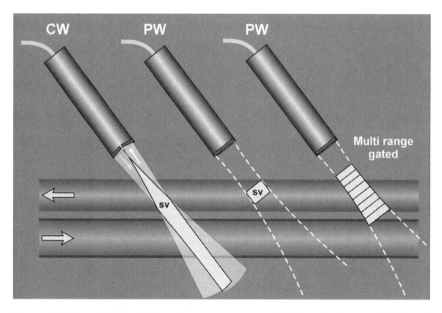

Figure 6. Schematic illustration of continuous wave (CW), pulsed wave (PW), and multirange-gated pulsed wave Doppler techniques. CW Dopplers contain 2 piezo-electric crystals: one continuously emits ultrasound while the other continuously detects ultrasound echoes from the tissue. The overlap field is the location where Doppler signals may be detected, sample volume (SV). The sample volume is smaller in PW Dopplers, and the SV depth may be selected (see text). In multirange gated PW Dopplers, the SV is sectioned, enabling identification of various Doppler spectra through the cross-section of the vessel.

longer, because of the longer time needed for the sound wave to reach the target area and return to the transducer. In turn, this increases the time between the pulses, i.e., reduces PRF, and thereby reduces the limit where aliasing occurs. To correctly detect very high velocities at large depths, for instance, in mitral stenoses, it may be necessary to switch to CW to avoid aliasing problems.

Doppler Flowmeter

In Doppler flowmeters, the mean blood velocity (cm/sec) is multiplied by the internal cross-sectional area (cm^2) to obtain the calculated volume blood flow (mL/min). This calculation is made automatically by some flowmeters by a multirange-gated ultrasonic beam where diameter is derived, or the flow is obtained semiautomatically with an online analog calculation unit where the internal diameter is manually inserted. In both techniques the accuracy of the calculated volume flow is highly dependent on correct determination of diameter because the error is squared at the calculation ($Q = v \cdot \pi \cdot r^2$), where v is velocity and r is the internal radius of the vessel. For example, if the radius of an artery of 3.0 mm is erroneously taken as 3.5 mm, the calculated blood flow is overestimated by 35%.

To minimize errors associated with angle insonation and vessel diameter, the transducer may be fixed to the vessel wall with a special cuff,[23] or by customizing special transducers with inbuilt angle correction (Fig. 7). Doppler flowmetry has the advantages over the electromagnetic flowmeter of requiring no zeroing and it is virtually unaffected by the vessel wall provided no air is entrapped within the wall material, for instance at newly inserted expanded PTFE and Dacron grafts. This problem might

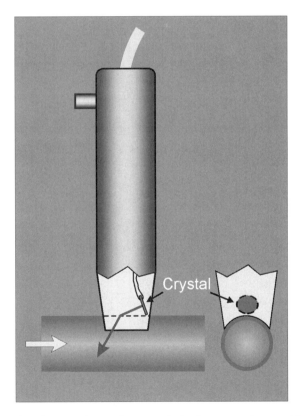

Figure 7. Doppler ultrasound transducer made for intraoperative use (developed by the author). The concave tip ensures good contact with the vessel wall even without a coupling medium. The transducer is placed at 90° to the vessel with the direction identifier at the top pointing upstream. The inbuilt crystal angle correction ensures fixed vessel insonation at 45°.

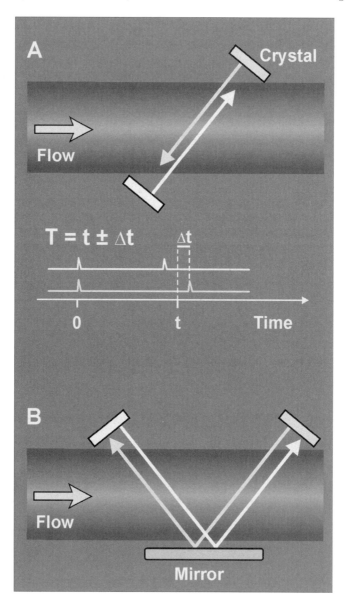

Figure 8. The principle of transit time flowmetry (**A**). Ultrasound is alternatingly sent upstream (yellow) and downstream (white). When blood is not flowing the passage time (T) is t. The passage time is minutely (Δt) increased when sent upstream and reduced by the same amount when sent downstream. The magnitude of Δt is dependent on blood flow. In practice, the transducer crystals are placed on the same side and the ultrasound beam is reflected at a mirror (dual pass)(**B**).

be reduced by gently squeezing the PTFE graft between 2 fingers for 2–5 minutes, enabling blood to penetrate the porous graft material.[24]

Transit Time Flowmeter

The most recently developed technique is the transit time flowmeter, which also uses ultrasound but not the Doppler principle. This method is based on the fact that ultrasound traveling against the bloodstream will take a longer time than when moving downstream (Fig. 8A). The theoretical basis for this technique has been known for some time, but it is only in the last decade that practical solutions have been available. An example is the Medi-Stim Butterfly flowmeter (Fig. 9) (Medi-Stim, Oslo, Norway), comprising a computer-based system with trend functions and ability to measure peripheral vascular resistance. Transit time flowmeters are very accurate, even at minute flow rates, and possess high zero line stability.

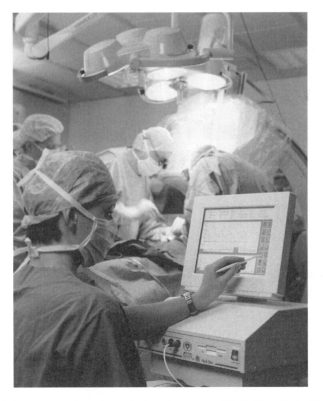

Figure 9. A computer-based transit time flowmeter (Medi-Stim, Oslo, Norway).

A practical transducer design is shown in Figures 8B and 10, where the 2 ultrasound crystals are placed on one side of the vessel and a metal reflector on the opposite side. This induces 2-fold passage of ultrasound through the blood vessels. The downstream crystal transmits a pulse of ultrasound to the upstream crystal. The difference in transit time propagation depends on the volume blood flow. The blood flow prolongs the time for the ultrasound beam to pass through the vessel against the bloodstream and a phase detector senses the time difference. A new sound beam is sent downstream and reflected. The blood flow decreases the transit time because the transmitting medium is also moving downstream. The process is then reversed several hundred times a second. Since the position of the crystals is fixed, the difference in transit time between the 2 directions can be related directly to volume blood flow. An extremely sensitive and stable detecting device is required to measure the very small difference between the transit times, which is on the order of picoseconds (10^{-12} sec), but the method has the advantage that the flow direction, as well as the volume flow, is indicated. A prerequisite for correct flow estimate is even insonation of the cross-section of the vessel. On the other hand, the difference in the transit times is dependent only on the moving particles in the vessel, thus making the measurements independent of the inner diameter.

At our hospital, the use of intraoperative flowmetry has been implemented in peripheral vascular procedures for about 35 years. In this pe-

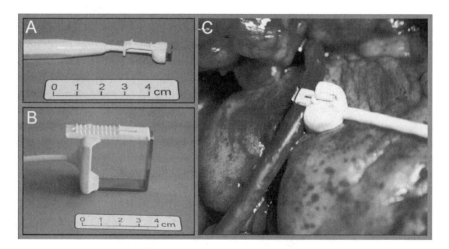

Figure 10. The 2 piezoelectric crystals of transit time transducers are placed within the housing on one side of the vessel, with a metal reflector on the opposite side. **A.** Transducer for small-caliber vessels, e.g., coronary bypasses, and for large vessels, e.g., aorta (**B**). **C.** Measurement of blood flow in a saphenous vein coronary bypass.

riod, all of the described techniques have been used. In the 1960s and 1970s, electromagnetic flowmetry was used, in the 1980s ultrasound Doppler technique with custom-made perioperative transducers were used, and in the 1990s we shifted to transit time flowmetry, which we regard as the method of choice for perioperative blood flow measurement.

Intra-Arterial Pressure Recording

Arteriography alone may be inadequate in the prediction of the hemodynamic significance of lesions, particularly in the aortoiliac region as reported by Sumner and Strandness.[25] The study noted that up to 30% of patients who had combined aortoiliac and femoropopliteal disease did not show hemodynamic improvement after a proximal reconstruction. This confirmed the inadequacy of arteriography alone in predicting the outcome of a proximal arterial reconstruction such as an aortobifemoral bypass in patients with multisegmental atherosclerosis.

Most investigators have generally agreed that any attempt to predict hemodynamic significance of a stenosis must be verified by direct intra-arterial pressure measurements.[26] Normally, the systolic pressure gradient between the aorta and the common femoral artery is below 10 mm Hg. In cases with unclear angiographic findings and a gradient below 10 mm Hg, intra-arterial papaverine is given, leading to a transient vasodilatation and increase in flow. Administration of papaverine is designed to mimic the flow increase seen with exercise. A systolic pressure gradient of more than 20 mm Hg is considered to be hemodynamically significant.[27]

There is little doubt that combined intra-arterial pressure and arteriography are extremely useful for documenting the hemodynamic status of an arterial segment. It has been suggested that these measurements must be done when stenotic lesions are found and angioplasty is being contemplated.[26] Furthermore, the pressure gradient should also be measured after completion of the dilatation to document the immediate result.

When reference pressure is obtained at the arm, great care should be taken when interpreting the data. Carter has shown that large systolic pressure wave amplification in the peripheral vessels may exist, especially in body cooling.[28,29] Therefore, if brachial or, even worse, radial pressure is taken to represent central prestenotic pressure, an overestimation of that pressure may be significant. Hence, the pressure gradient over the stenosis may be overestimated. This effect is reduced when the body is kept warm to induce peripheral vasodilatation.

When pressure is recorded during angiography, a "pull-through" technique should be applied whenever possible. The pressure transducer catheter line is introduced and moved proximal to the obstruction to measure the preobstruction pressure. Then the catheter is pulled through the obstruction to obtain the postobstruction pressure. The difference between these pressures indicates the degree of obstruction.

It is uncommon for patients with critical limb ischemia to get significant relief following reconstructing of the profunda femoris artery only. However, in cases where there is occlusion of the first part of the profunda artery, it may be worthwhile to reopen this artery. One cannot expect significant improvement of symptoms unless there is a marked pressure gradient between external iliac/common femoral artery and the peripheral part of the profunda femoris artery, for instance on the order of at least 20 mm Hg at rest.

Measurement of Vascular Outflow Resistance

Following femorodistal bypass surgery, both limb salvage rate and graft patency are dependent on outflow resistance. Preoperative arteriographic visualization of these vessels does not inform us of whether their functional capacity is adequate to keep a distal bypass open. Studies have shown that intraoperative measurements of distal resistance are predictive in terms of outcome of femorodistal bypasses.[30–32] Some authors have defined a sharp cutoff point above which femorodistal grafts are prone to reocclude.[31] Attempts have been made to define a level of resistance above which primary amputation should be performed instead of arterial reconstruction,[33] or levels where reopening of the graft can be neglected in case reocclusion occurs in the early postoperative phase. However, factors such as the nature of the infused fluid, the tone of the peripheral vascular tree, etc., may significantly influence the results.[33,34] Peripheral resistance is defined as mean arterial pressure divided by mean arterial flow, and is often expressed in peripheral resistance units (PRU), mm Hg $\times$ min $\times$ mL^{-1}.

Outflow resistance (R) has been examined with different techniques, one of which is the basic *pressure (P)* divided by *flow (Q)* measurement, which represents the definition of vascular resistance (R = P / Q). This technique was simplified, as described by Ascer and co-workers.[31] A mathematical rewriting simplifies the equation to include the pressure integral when a fixed volume (V) is injected into the distal artery (Fig. 11). In this technique, flowmetry is not needed, as a special pressure integration unit is used.

Recently, noninvasive techniques examining outflow vessels preoperatively have been presented. The most promising is the pulse-generated runoff (PGR) where a pressure cuff is placed around the calf or thigh and Doppler examination of the calf (or foot) vessels is performed after rapid repetitive inflations of the cuff.[35,36] The method has a semiquantitative scoring system. With the technique, a standardized artificial arterial pres-

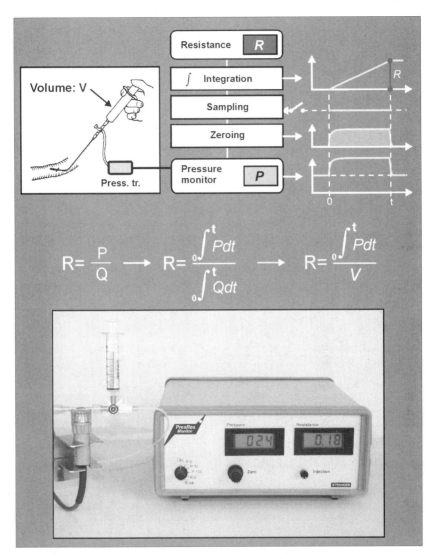

Figure 11. Outflow resistance measurement by the pressure integral technique. The mathematical basis is shown in the equation. Vascular resistance (R) is by definition the mean pressure (P) divided by mean blood flow (Q), for instance, the pressure increase when a volume is injected by a syringe. This expression may be integrated as shown in the middle equation. However, as the time integral of flow is equal to the injected volume in that time period (V), the middle equation is reduced to constitute the pressure integral divided by a fixed volume. In the unit shown below (PresRes Monitor, developed by the author), the vascular outflow resistance is obtained by pressure recording during infusion, subtracted from backpressure (zeroing), sampled during a fixed infusion time (infusion flow 100 mL/min) and automatically integrated during that time.

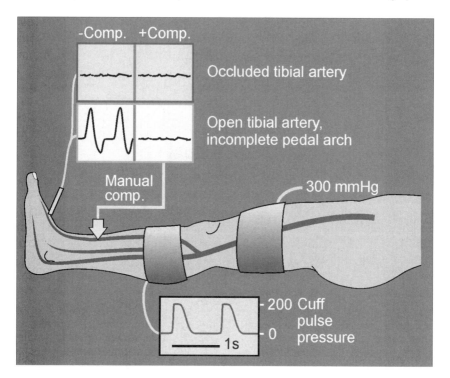

Figure 12. Schematic presentation of the noninvasive pulse-generated runoff technique for evaluating outflow vessels prior to surgery. A proximal occlusion cuff prevents interference from the proximal arterial pulse. A pressure cuff placed at the calf level is intermittently inflated to produce artificial pressure/flow waves, which may be detected in the distal branches when the artery is open (lower left curve). The pedal arch is examined by manually compressing (+Comp.) the leg arteries as described by Scott and co-workers.[37]

sure wave is created in the calf, and detected in the leg arteries by Doppler ultrasound technique. The latest refinement of the procedure includes a pedal arch patency test (Fig. 12). This test, applied to all 3 leg arteries, may predict the likelihood for a femorodistal bypass to remain open, and could be of help to select patients where a primary amputation should be considered.[37]

Anatomical Tests

Intraoperative Arteriography

Intraoperative arteriography is regarded the "gold standard" for control of infrainguinal reconstruction, either by conventional arteriography or digital subtraction arteriography. It has been shown that technical defects may be observed in more than 20% of the cases.[38] Due to the direct visualization of the vessels, interpretation of the findings is generally easy. By detecting defects during the operation, they can be corrected, thereby improving the patency rate. However, this method has a few disadvantages. Usually only the graft and the distal anastomosis are visualized, which is unfortunate since technical defects may also be located at the upper anastomosis. The arteriograms are normally taken in one plane only, and small defects may be hidden in the contrast material. The method includes injection of contrast material, which may lead to allergic reactions, and may be nephrotoxic.

Angioscopy

Following the introduction of modern fiberoptic angioscopes, a visualization of the graft and the anastomotic area can be obtained. Angioscopy may be used to detect residual valvular flaps, which may be retained following in situ vein bypass grafting (Fig. 13). This method can also be combined with endovascular closure of venous side branches, and in evaluating venous valves. In some areas, angioscopy is superior to arteriography. Neville and co-workers[39] found in an in vivo model that planar arteriography in one projection identified 60% of the arterial intimal flaps, while angioscopy and intravascular ultrasound visualized all of them. Comparing angioscopy with arteriography, the latter method is especially inferior in identifying thrombi; sometimes arteriography underestimates or misses mural or retained thrombi and debris.[40]

A disadvantage of angioscopy is that it does not allow visualization of the outflow arteries including the pedal arch, whereas angiography visually includes these arteries. Furthermore, only anatomical details may be shown, and no impression of peripheral vascular resistance is obtained. Sometimes clear visualization is difficult due to bleeding from side branches and the method may be technically difficult to perform. The equipment is expensive, especially disposable angioscopes, and there may be difficulties with cleaning and sterilization.

Color Flow Duplex Scanning

Color flow duplex scanning is a direct noninvasive technique and includes 3 modalities: real-time *B-mode* (brightness mode) image, *Doppler velocity spectrum* (usually PW), and *color-coded flow information* of blood velocity superimposed the B-mode image. The technique provides both

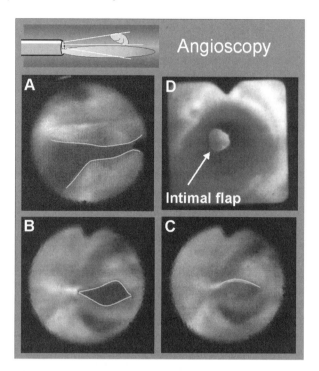

Figure 13. Angioscopy images from venous (**A-C**) and arterial (**D**) investigations. **A.** Incompetent venous valve with floppy cusps that do not approximate during Valsalva maneuver. The same valve after successful angioscopically guided external valvulo- plasty, during opening (**B**) and closing (**C**). The images are retained from a video se- quence, hence the somewhat reduced image quality. For the benefit of clarity, the edges of the valve cusps are artificially outlined. **D.** A residual intimal flap after arte- rial reconstruction.

anatomical and physiological information, and has become the key in- strument in vascular laboratories.

Preoperative and Postoperative Evaluation

Color coding has the advantage over plain duplex (B-mode + spectral Doppler) of enabling rapid identification of arteries, and specifically areas of stenoses and obstructions with flow disturbances. Atherosclerotic plaques are identified by the presence of calcification or increased echogenicity. Stenoses can be detected by using different criteria, such as peak systolic velocity (PSV) within the narrowing, the ratio of PSV in the stenosis to PSV in a normal segment close to it, end-diastolic velocity or, more subjectively, by noting the degree of spectral broadening. Several studies indicate a high degree of accuracy in assessment of the aortoiliac and femoropopliteal arteries, but slightly poorer accuracy in distal arteries.[41] Most centers use a PSV ratio greater than 2.0 as a stenosis criterion for detecting a stenosis larger than 50% diameter reduction. These studies have challenged arteriography as the "gold standard" for the evaluation of lower extremity atherosclerosis, especially in the aortoiliac and femoropopliteal arteries. Consequently, an increasing number of hospitals now base the selection of therapy on color flow duplex investigations. For planning femorodistal reconstructions, most surgeons will find duplex scanning not optimal, and regard arteriography a prerequisite.

Deep vessels, low blood velocities, calcified plaque with acoustic shadows, and bowel gas frequently reduce the quality of the color flow duplex scanning and sometimes make it inconclusive. Software enhancement, for example, power mode Doppler based on signal intensity rather than the Doppler shift, increases sensitivity and may be used to improve locating vessels with low blood flow states or improve delineation of hypoechoic plaques. Furthermore, echo enhancers (ultrasound contrast), administered intravenously, may significantly improve the investigation in problem areas such as in the pelvic, distal thigh (Hunter's canal), and calf arteries.

Duplex scanning provides tissue images in multiple planes on the operating table, together with a velocity profile analysis for evaluation of the hemodynamic results. Color codification of the blood velocity placed on the tissue image gives additional global, 2-dimensional representation of the flow patterns in vessels, anastomoses, and grafts.[42] Furthermore, anatomical defects such as loose intimal flaps, strictures, intraluminal thrombi, loose debris, residual stenosis, and misplaced sutures may be identified[43] (Fig. 14). Flow abnormalities found with Doppler spectral analysis or Doppler color coding helps to identify significant lesions.[44] According to published reports on intraoperative use of duplex ultrasound for assessment of reconstructive vascular surgery, defects are found in 20–30%. Only 5–10% of these are judged as significant and consequently corrected. The indications for vessel reentry are subjective and empirical. The decision to revise a reconstruction is based principally on the basis of the surgeon's judgment that the residual anatomical defect or hemodynamic disturbance may cause complications.

Intraoperatively, the working conditions for the sonographer, which in most cases is the surgeon, are poor. The need for sterile conditions necessitates that a technician operate the scanner somewhat remotely from the surgical field. Sometimes it may be difficult to maintain control of both the investigated blood vessel and the monitor. Perhaps these problems could be reduced if a color liquid crystal display (LCD) were available, attached to the top of the transducer (Fig. 15), and the scanner controls operated by voice recognition, merely ordering the command.

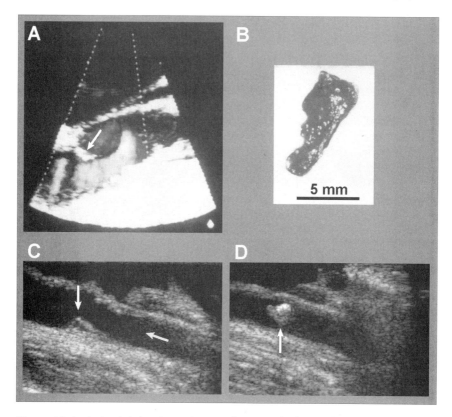

Figure 14. An intimal defect (arrow) protruding into the lumen following carotid endarterectomy (CEA), as detected by color duplex scanning (**A**). At reintervention, an intimal flap of 2 × 7 mm was identified and removed (**B**). **C.** B-mode image of a residual intimal flap detected following CEA (white arrow). Yellow arrow indicates direction of blood flow. After revising the defect, a new examination identified a fresh thrombus (**D**, arrow), at the site where an arterial clamp was applied during the first revision. Consequently, a second reopening was necessary. (The images were kindly provided by O.D. Saether (A and B) and T. Dahl (C and D), Trondheim University Hospital, Norway.)

Intravascular Ultrasound (IVUS)

For endovascular procedures, intravascular (intraluminal) ultrasound may be the method of choice, since it can visualize the composition of the lesion and thereby help to select the proper treatment modality. Furthermore, residual plaques or flaps can be detected, and a sufficient stent wall contact can be confirmed.[45] The technique will earn more attention when combined with *therapy constitution*. A single introduction, therapeutical IVUS unit with a percutaneous transluminal angioplasty (PTA) balloon, which could be reality in the future, is hypothesized in Figure 16. As microcatheter technology is being refined, one might expect that addition of dual pressure sensors and a Doppler ultrasound transducer at the tip should not raise the catheter cost significantly. With the pressure sensors, indicated as P1 and P2, the pressure gradient is measured continuously to evaluate the immediate effect of angioplasty. These entities are already available on separate units; miniaturized pressure sensors are available in angiography guidewires (e.g., Cardiometrics WaveWire, Endosonics, San Diego, CA, USA), as are Doppler ultrasound transducers (e.g., Cardiometrics FloMap, Endosonics, San Diego, CA, USA). Combined IVUS/PTA catheters are already available (e.g., MegaSonics F/X and OTW PTCA catheters, Endosonics, San Diego, CA, USA).

Three-Dimensional (3D) Mode

Vascular disorders are essentially 3-dimensional and should logically be visualized that way, especially in regard to vascular malformations and the quantification of atherosclerotic plaques.[46,47] Current technology has been used for 3D rendering of larger organs such as the heart and kidney, and volume estimation of abdominal organs.[48,49] In particular, 3D

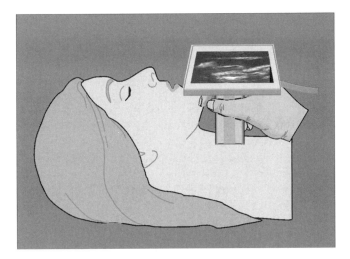

Figure 15. Suggested solution for the problem of keeping visual contact with the monitor when the ultrasound scanner is located somewhat remotely apart from the surgical field to preserve sterile conditions. A color liquid crystal display (in sterile transparent wrappings) might be attached to the top of the transducer enabling direct visualization of the vessel below. Scanner controls should be operated by voice recognition, by merely ordering the command.

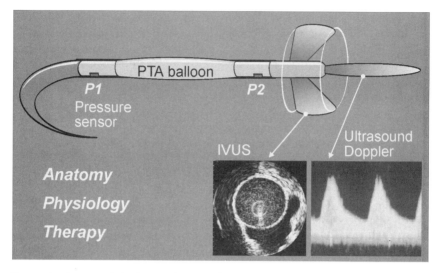

Figure 16. Suggested single introduction, therapeutical IVUS unit with a PTA balloon that might be available in the future. This combines description of intraluminal *anatomy* (IVUS), *physiology* (pressure gradient [P2-P1], and Doppler ultrasound) and *therapy* (PTA with/without stent) in one introduction procedure.

echocardiography has proved to offer important additional clinical information.[50–54]

3D/4D Representation

A 2D ultrasound image is composed of $X \cdot Y$ picture elements, or *pixels* (Fig. 17). This concept can be extended to the imaging of 3D objects. The depth, or Z dimension, can be modeled by stacking a series of 2D planes in depth. The 2D picture elements are then interpolated to become cubes. These cubes, which form the 3D image, are called volume elements, or *voxels*. The volume representation is called a *cuberille*. When volumetric information is correlated with time to form the 4th dimension (4D), every voxel element has variations over time. Representation in 4D is particularly used when time dynamics plays an essential role, e.g., displaying the heart or cardiovascular structures over a cardiac cycle.

At present, the process of making 3D images based on ultrasonography is divided into 4 steps (Fig. 18):

- data acquisition and filtering
- volume generation
- data processing
- visualization.

Several methods are available to acquire 2D images to be transformed to 3D data. The region of interest may be insonated by movement of the probe, by rotating, tilting, or linear translation. When the position sensor system is applied, for instance, based on magnetic tracking of the scanhead, the transducer may be moved about freely to generate the set of 2D images that are transformed into the 3D domain.[55] In the future, 2D array transducers will probably be used to a greater degree. Extremely high pro-

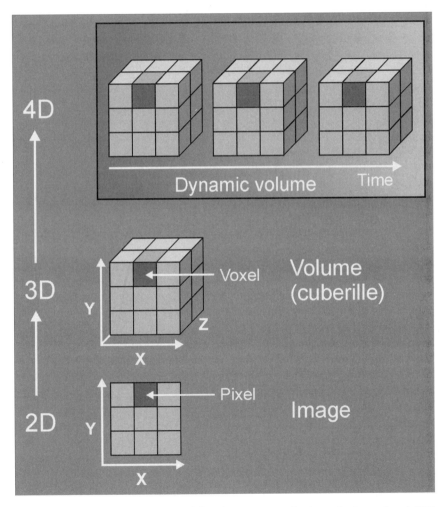

Figure 17. Schematic illustration of the elements constituting a 2-dimensional (2D) ultrasound image, an image volume (3D), and a dynamic volume (4D), displaying volumetric information over time. The basic element in 2D is a pixel, whereas it is a voxel in 3D/4D.

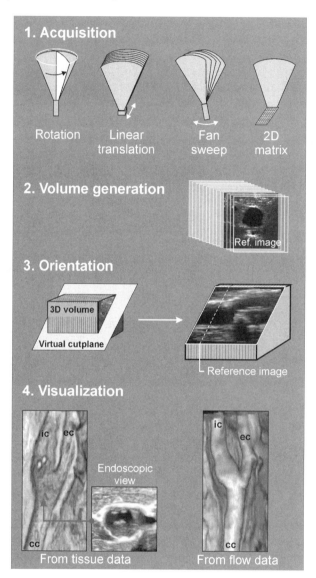

Figure 18. Ultrasonic 3D acquisition (**1**) and post-processing (**2–4**). (**1**). A 3D image volume is created by translation of the ultrasound transducer, by rotation, linear translation, or fan sweep. When the position sensor system is applied, the transducer may be moved about freely to generate the set of 2D images. In the future, 2D matrix transducers most probably will be used. (**2**). Volume generation. A series of 2D sections are placed one behind the other to form an image volume. A reference image is chosen within this series where important clinical information is displayed. (**3–4**): Visualization of the region of interest within the image volume is done with virtual cutplanes (viewing planes) in any direction and location within the volume. These cutplanes may be freely moved and rotated at any angle. The cutplanes are slices in the image volume and visualized as images based on either tissue or flow data (**4**).

cessing speeds and capacities are needed, however, for near real-time 3D display. The acquisition may involve respiration- and ECG-triggering to reduce movement artifacts.

During 3D data acquisition and image processing, the data undergo several transformation and filtering operations. The first post-processing step is to transform the 2D video-captured data into a cubic representation of the image volume by interpolating neighboring pixels in the 2D video capture.

The next post-processing step, orientation, applies to the interactive process of reviewing the data when "viewing" windows are opened for examining the volume. This viewing function is the essential tool for the positioning of viewing planes in relation to objects or structures that are of clinical interest.

The final phase of post-processing is the computation of 3D/4D images containing information of tissue surfaces, their orientation, and distance from the viewing plane. Surface points that are more distant from the observer will become darker than points that are close to the observer. Our studies on vascular 3D processing[56] indicate that gradient shading is an applicable and robust technique. In gradient shading, the orientation of surface together with distance determines the gray value, providing images with visual appearance correlating well with normal photographic techniques. Figure 19 depicts the proximal anastomosis of a patient with a reversed vein femoropopliteal bypass applying the 3D gradient-shading technique.

Color Doppler velocity or power energy mode data have been used to isolate vascular structures from gray scale tissue images, thereby obtaining a clearer view of the vessel anatomy.[56-58] The use of velocity or power mode data has a 2-fold advantage over gray scale-generated images. First, a major difficulty with volume data visualization is that the majority of volume elements do not contain clinically relevant data. Extraction of clinically useful information may therefore be difficult other than when displaying a 2D slice. Using flow information reduces this problem. Second, eliminating the gray scale and instead using flow data for surface rendering also improves visualization of vascular structures (Fig. 20). This is especially important when understanding complex spatial relationships.

Three-dimensional representation of the vasculature may become a valuable adjunct to conventional 2D imaging. An advantage of 3D representation lies in the fact that orientations are preserved, enabling descriptive data not definable by 2D formats or a verbal report to be conveyed rapidly and effectively to the clinician. This may allow physicians with less experience to interpret complex images and make diagnostic decisions that currently require specialists in sonography. The effectiveness of this transfer of information, however, depends on how realistic the 3D images appear.

Mathematical modeling may be applied to the acquired dataset to calculate volume of structures.[49] The Vingmed EchoPac 3D (GE Vingmed Sound, Horten, Norway) allows different acquisition modes and is computer platform-independent. Interactive contouring does the volume

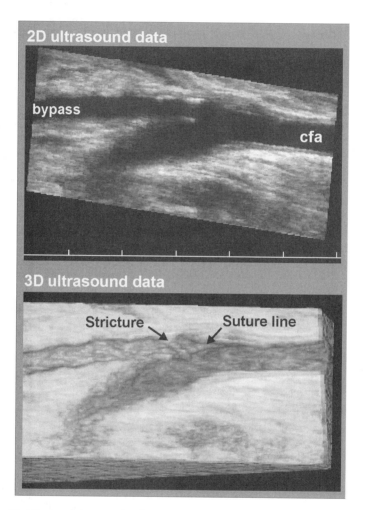

Figure 19. Views of the proximal anastomosis of a patient with a reversed vein femoropopliteal bypass (bypass) to the common femoral artery (cfa), applying 3D gradient-shading technique. The 3D image is generated from the longitudinal reference image at the top and subsequently underlying parallel planes (in depth). The arrows point to the suture line of the anastomosis, and what is supposed to be a wall stricture.

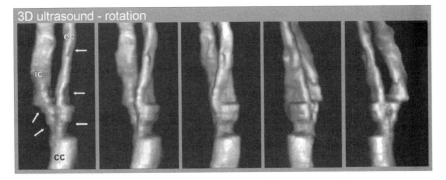

Figure 20. Sections from rotation of a 3D rendering of a carotid bifurcation. The images are based on power mode Doppler data. Tissue data is suppressed by reducing the tissue gain level. The arrows point to irregularities of the flow contour, coinciding with stenotic parts of the vessels. cc = common carotid artery; ic = internal carotid; ec = external carotid arteries.

modeling, and the volume calculations have proven very accurate. An example is shown in Figure 21.

Our experience shows that 3D/4D ultrasound is superior to 2D in communicating volumetric information, and the use of ultrasound power energy mode may overcome problems related to poor B-mode visualization. Clinically, 3D imaging may become important in relation to arterial reconstructions performed without angiography, e.g., carotid endarterectomies or even beating heart coronary surgery in the future.

Examples of Flowmetry in Peripheral Vascular Disease

Detection of Side Branches During In Situ Bypass Surgery

At in situ bypass surgery, the side branches of the great saphenous vein must be interrupted to prevent them from becoming arteriovenous fistulae after the reconstruction. Following completion of the proximal and distal anastomoses, vessel clamps are removed and blood flow through the bypass is established. Major tributaries of the vein can be visually identified and ligated without difficulty. However, smaller branches often have to be detected by other means, mainly intraoperative flowmetry, in order to avoid major surgical dissection. It is important to locate these residual fistulae since they may cause graft failure.[59]

The detection of arteriovenous connections has a qualitative aim; exact blood flow values are less relevant. A flow probe of appropriate size is placed around the vein, just below the proximal anastomosis. When using

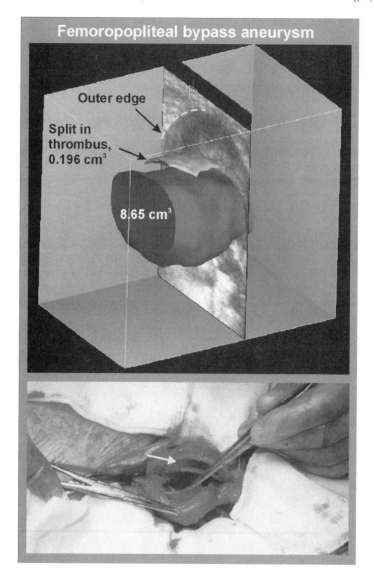

Figure 21. Calculating volume of a femoropopliteal bypass aneurysm using the Vingmed Echopac 3D. The central gray volume (with the annotation 8.65 cm^3) is the demarcation of the open flow section of the aneurysm. The section above is a split in the thrombus, verified at surgical removal of the aneurysm (arrow). The outer edge of the vessel wall is indicated by the interrupted line.

transit time flowmetry, either sterile saline or ultrasound gel is used to maintain acoustic coupling between the probe and measuring site. Pulsatile flow curves will immediately appear on the display (Fig. 22). The vein is occluded, manually or by means of an atraumatic clamp, successively at different sites along its course, from the transducer to the distal anastomosis.

Reverberating flow profile, indicating no net blood flow (Fig. 22, position 1), is found when there is no leakage flow between the transducer and the compression site. If flow is detected during clamping, we can expect to find an open side branch proximal to the site of clamping (Fig. 22, position 2) that can subsequently be ligated.

Intraoperative Functional Evaluation of a Vascular Reconstruction

As distal femorotibial bypass grafting has become more common, supplementary methods are necessary for intraoperative control. The primary aim is to obtain information on the prognosis for the immediate re-

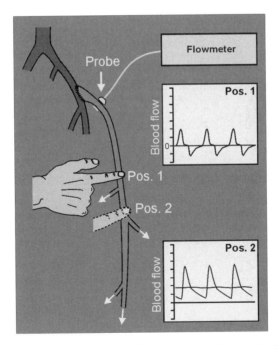

Figure 22. Procedure for detection of side branches during in situ bypass surgery. During the examination, the finger is compressing the artery. If net flow is detected, the finger is downstream a side branch acting as arteriovenous fistula. This is subsequently ligated.

sult of the reconstruction. Several studies have shown that perioperative flow values have prognostic values.[1,3] The risk of early postoperative occlusion is significantly increased if the basal blood flow after femoropopliteal reconstruction is less than 100 mL/min or the papaverine-induced flow (intra-arterial injection of 40 mg papaverine) is less than 200 mL/min (Fig. 23). The effect of papaverine is reduced if the surgery is

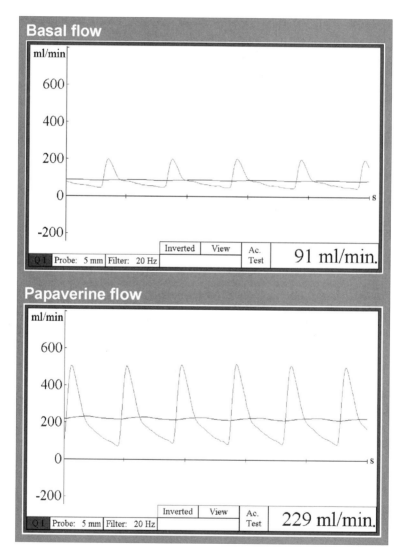

Figure 23. Mean and pulsatile blood flow curves in a successful femoropopliteal bypass. Upper panel: Basal flow. Lower panel: Following intra-arterial injection of papaverine.

performed under epidural anesthesia, since basal flow is already increased.

Obviously, blood flow values do not necessarily provide information about anatomical aberrations due to technical failure. Ideally, intraoperative arteriography or B-mode scanning is performed in order to supply the surgeon with an anatomical evaluation as well.

Cost Effectiveness

In the future, it is likely that health economy will be even more constrained than today. Cost effectiveness of intraoperative methods will therefore have to be evaluated thoroughly before they are introduced into the clinical routine. The selection of methods will be based on the number of reconstructions performed by the institution each year, and the economic situation of the hospital. Furthermore, the procedure must be easy to use and should not prolong the operating time unduly.

The costs of the procedures must be weighed against the possibility of leaving a less satisfactory reconstruction. In the long run, this could lead to graft occlusion with amputation as a result in patients with critical limb ischemia (CLI).[60,61] Initially, the cost of amputation is similar to vascular reconstructions, but the patient with an amputation may be a burden on society for many years. Consequently, efforts to improve patency rate of reconstructions for CLI can be regarded as good economy.

The Future

Angiography is one of the cornerstones of intraoperative diagnostics in critical limb ischemia, and in many centers it is regarded as part of the minimum facilities needed for the management of these patients. Angioscopy still has to be evaluated as far as the efficiency of detecting significant failures are concerned. These methods will probably supplement each other in the near future.

Further refinements in 3D rendering of the vessels are anticipated, especially in ultrasound techniques. Therapeutic IVUS catheters with pressure transducers and Doppler ultrasound for PTA and stent insertion will probably also emerge. Real-time 3D ultrasound scanners require a fast computer kernel and new transducer technology, probably a crystal matrix design. With such technology, a 3D representation of blood flow and flow vectors may enhance our perception of local flow conditions and morphological changes in diseased states. Along that line of evolution, we hope that color maps for energy dissipation are developed and implemented to directly locate and visualize the hemodynamic importance of arterial obstructions.

Resistance measurements will probably have a more important place in this area in the future. Patients who end up with an amputation after vascular surgery have often undergone 2 to 4 attempts of revascularization prior to amputation. Thus, a key problem is to decide when to do a primary amputation, or when to give the patient one chance of reconstruction, and then stay away from a second attempt in case reocclusion occurs. Finally, resistance measurements can perhaps give us some idea of when it will be feasible to perform a femorodistal bypass graft to the leg arteries. Reliable data concerning cutoff values are warranted.

Two basic functional tests are going to persist: flowmetry and intra-arterial pressure measurements. For flowmeters, transit time technology will probably be chosen because of its accuracy and ease of handling. When combined, these measurements constitute outflow resistance.

References

1. Dedichen H. Hemodynamics in arterial reconstructions of the lower limb: blood flow. Acta Chir Scand 1976; 142:213–220.
2. Stranden E, Myhre HO. Intraoperative diagnostics in critical limb ischaemia. Critical Ischaemia 1994; 4(2):44–52.
3. Dedichen H. The papaverine test for blood flow potential of ilio-femoral arteries. Acta Chir Scand 1976; 142:107–113.
4. Hickey NC, Shearman CP, Crowson MC, et al. Iloprost improves femoro-distal graft flow after a single bolus injection. Eur J Vasc Surg 1991; 5:19–22.
5. Smith FCT, Shearman CP. Pharmacological manipulation of peripheral resistance during distal vascular reconstruction. VASA 1992; 36(suppl):55–57.
6. Cappelen C Jr, Efskind L, Hall KV. Electromagnetic flowmeter measurements of the blood flow in the ascending aorta during cardiac surgery. Acta Chir Scand 1966; 356B(suppl):129–133.
7. Cappelen C Jr, Hall KV. Electromagnetic blood flowmetry in clinical surgery. Acta Chir Scand 1967; 368(suppl):3–27.
8. Cronestrand R, Ekestrom S, Hambraeus G. The value of blood flow measurements in acute arterial surgery. Scand J Thorac Cardiovasc Surg 1969; 3(1):48–51.
9. Cappelen C Jr, Hall KV. Intra-operative blood flow measurements with electromagnetic flowmeter. Prog Surg 1970; 8:102–123.
10. Semb GS, Cappelen C Jr, Hall KV, Efskind L. Postoperative aortic regurgitation related to perioperative blood flowmetry in ball valve replacement. Scand J Thorac Cardiovasc Surg 1970; 4(1):25–30.
11. Hall KV, Fjeld NB. Perioperative assessment of run-off by electromagnetic flowmetry. Scand J Clin Lab Invest 1973; 128(suppl):185–188.
12. Foxworthy JV, Monro JL, Lewis B. The response to papaverine in coronary artery bypass graft flows. J Cardiovasc Surg 1985; 26:439–442.
13. Walpoth BH, Bosshard A, Genyk I, Kipfer B, Berdat PA, et al. Transit-time flow measurement for detection of early graft failure during myocardial revascularization. Ann Thorac Surg 1998; 66:1097–1100.
14. Walpoth BH, Bosshard A, Kipfer B, Berdat PA, Althaus U, et al. Failed coronary artery bypass anastomosis detected by intraoperative coronary flow measurement. Eur J Cardiothorac Surg 1998; 14(suppl 1):S76–S81.

15. D'Ancona G, Karamanoukian HL, Salerno TA, Schmid RN, Bergsland J. Flow measurement in coronary surgery. Heart Surg Forum 1999; 2(2):121–124.
16. Geddes LA, Baker LE. Principles of Applied Biomedical Instrumentation, 2nd ed. New York, John Wiley and Sons, 1975.
17. Sykes MK, Vickers MD, Hull CJ. Principles of Clinical Measurement. Oxford, Blackwell Scientific Publications, 1981.
18. Roberts VC. Haematocrit variations and electromagnetic flowmeter sensitivity. Biomed Eng 1969; 4(9):408–412.
19. Dennis J, Wyatt DG. Effect of hematocrit value upon electromagnetic flowmeter sensitivity. Circ Res 1969; 24(6):875–886.
20. Lundell A, Bergqvist D. Intraoperative flow measurements in vascular reconstruction. Ann Chir Gynaecol 1992; 81(2):187–191.
21. Angelsen B. Waves, signals and signal processing in medical ultrasonics. Dept. of Biomedical Engineering, University of Trondheim, 1991.
22. Hennerici MG, Neuerburg-Heusler D. Vascular Diagnosis with Ultrasound. Georg Thieme Verlag, 1997.
23. Beard JD, Evans JM, Skidmore R, Horrocks M. A Doppler flowmeter for use in theatre. Ultrasound Med Biol 1986; 12(11):883–889.
24. Rostad H, Grip A, Hall C. Blood flow measurement in PTFE grafts. J Cardiovasc Surg (Torino) 1987; 28(3):262–265.
25. Sumner DS, Strandness DE Jr. Aortoiliac reconstruction in patients with combined iliac and superficial femoral occlusion. Surgery 1977; 28:348–355.
26. Strandness DE Jr. Transluminal angioplasty: a surgeon's viewpoint. Am J Roentgenol 1980; 135:998–1000.
27. Thiele BL, Bandyk DF, Zierler RE. A systematic approach to the assessment of aortoiliac disease. Arch Surg 1983; 18:477–485.
28. Carter SA. Effect of age, cardiovascular disease, and vasomotor changes on transmission of arterial pressure waves through the lower extremities. Angiology 1978; 29:601–616.
29. Carter SA, Tate RB. The effect of body heating and cooling on the ankle and toe systolic pressures in arterial disease. J Vasc Surg 1992; 16:148–153.
30. Ascer E, Veith FJ, Morin L, et al. Quanitative assessment of outflow resistance in lower extremity arterial reconstruction. J Surg Res 1984; 37:8–15.
31. Ascer E, Veith FJ, White-Flores SA, et al. Intraoperative outflow resistance as a predictor of late patency of femoropopliteal and infrapopliteal bypasses. J Vasc Surg 1987; 5:820–827.
32. Beard ID, Scott DIA, Skidmore R, et al. Operative assessment of femorodistal bypass grafts using a new Doppler flowmeter. Br J Surg 1989; 76:925–928.
33. Parvin SD, Evans DH, Bell PRF. Peripheral pressure measurement in the assessment of severe peripheral vascular disease. Br J Surg 1985; 72:751–753.
34. Wahlberg E, Line PD, Olofsson P, Swedenborg J. Infusion methods for determination of peripheral resistance: influence of infused medium and back pressure. Ann Vasc Surg 1994; 8:172–178.
35. Beard JD, Scott DIA, Evans JM, et al. Pulse generated runoff (PGR): a new method of assessing calf vessel patency. Br J Surg 1988; 75:361–363.
36. Davies AH, Horrocks M. Outflow resistance measurements. Ann Chir Gynaecol 1992; 81(2):183–186.
37. Scott DJA, Horrocks EH, Kinsella D, Horrocks M. Preoperative assessment of the pedal arch using pulse generated runoff and subsequent femorodistal outcome. Eur J Vasc Surg 1994; 8:20–25.
38. Myhre HO, Kordt KF, Stranden E. Pre- and perioperative angiography and clinical physiological measurements. Acta Chir Scand 1987; 538:132–138.

39. Neville RF, Yasuhara H, Watanabe Bl, et al. Endovascular management of arterial intimal defects: an experimental comparison by arteriography, angioscopy, and intravascular ultrasonography. J Vasc Surg 1991; 13:496–502.
40. Segalowitz J, Grundfest WS, Treiman RL, et al. Angioscopy for intraoperative management of thromboembolectomy. Arch Surg 1990; 125:1357–1361.
41. Koelemay MJW, Hartog D, Prins MH, et al. Diagnosis of arterial disease of the lower extremity with duplex ultrasonography. Br J Surg 1996; 83:404–409.
42. Saether O, Mathisen S. Intraoperative Doppler. Ann Chir Gynaecol 1992; 81(2):176–177.
43. Myhre HO, Saether OD, Mathisen SR, Angelsen BAJ. Color coded duplex scanning during carotid endarterectomy. In Greenhalgh RM, Hollier LH (eds): Surgery for Stroke. London, WB Saunders, Ltd, pp 253–258, 1993.
44. Bandyk DF, Kaebnick HW, Adams MB, Towne JB. Turbulence occurring after carotid bifurcation endarterectomy: a harbinger of residual and recurrent stenosis. J Vasc Surg 1988; 7:261–274.
45. Pandian NG, Kreis A, Weintraub A, Kumar R. Intravascular ultrasound assessment of arterial dissection, intimal flaps, and intraarterial thrombi. Am J Cardiac Imaging 1991; 5(1):72–77.
46. Delcker A, Diener HC. Quantification of atherosclerotic plaques in carotid arteries by three-dimensional ultrasound. Br J Radiol 1994; 67;672–678.
47. Palombo C, Kozakova M, Morizzo C, Andreuccetti F, Tondini A, et al. Ultrafast three-dimensional ultrasound: application to carotid artery imaging. Stroke 1998; 29(8):1631–1637.
48. Gilja OH, Thune N, Matre K, Hausken T, Odegaard S, et al. In vitro evaluation of three-dimensional ultrasonography in volume estimation of abdominal organs. Ultrasound Med Biol 1994; 20:157–165.
49. Gilja OH, Hausken T, Berstad A, Odegaard S. Measurements of organ volume by ultrasonography. Proc Inst Mech Eng 1999; 213(3):247–259.
50. Pandian NG, Roelandt J, Nanda NC, Sugeng L, Cao QL, et al. Dynamic three-dimensional echocardiography: methods and clinical potential. Echocardiography 1994; 11:237–259.
51. De Castro S, Yao J, Fedele F, Pandian NG. Three-dimensional echocardiography in ischemic heart disease. Coron Artery Dis 1998; 9(7):427–434.
52. De Castro S, Yao J, Pandian NG. Three-dimensional echocardiography: clinical relevance and application. Am J Cardiol 1998; 81(12A):96G–102G.
53. Kardon RE, Cao QL, Masani N, Sugeng L, Supran S, et al. New insights and observations in three-dimensional echocardiographic visualization of ventricular septal defects: experimental and clinical studies. Circulation 1998; 98(13):1307–1314.
54. Acar P, Laskari C, Rhodes J, Pandian N, Warner K, et al. Three-dimensional echocardiographic analysis of valve anatomy as a determinant of mitral regurgitation after surgery for atrioventricular septal defects. Am J Cardiol 1999; 83(5):745–749.
55. Gilja OH, Hausken T, Olafsson S, Matre K, Odegaard S. In vitro evaluation of three-dimensional ultrasonography based on magnetic scanhead tracking. Ultrasound Med Biol 1998; 24(8):1161–1167.
56. Stranden E, Slagsvold C-E, Morken B, Alker HJ, Bjørdal J. Three-dimensional ultrasound visualization of peripheral vessels. In Greenhalgh RM (ed): Vascular Imaging for Surgeons. London, WB Saunders Co Ltd, pp 71–80, 1995.
57. Pretorius DH, Nelson TR, Jaffe JS. 3-Dimensional sonographic analysis based on color flow Doppler and gray scale image data: a preliminary report. J Ultrasound Med 1992; 11:225–232.

58. Li X, Shiota T, Delabays A, Teien D, Zhou X, et al. Flow convergence flow rates from 3-dimensional reconstruction of color Doppler flow maps for computing transvalvular regurgitant flows without geometric assumptions: an in vitro quantitative flow study. J Am Soc Echocardiogr 1999; 12(12):1035–1044.
59. Donaldson MC, Mannick JA, Whittemore AD. Causes of primary graft failure after in situ saphenous vein bypass grafting. J Vasc Surg 1992; 15:113–120.
60. Mackey WC, McCullough JL, Conlon TP, et al. The costs of surgery for limb-threatening ischemia. Surgery 1986; 99:26–35.
61. Raviola CA, Nichter LS, Baker JD, et al. Cost of treating advanced leg ischemia. Arch Surg 1988; 123:495–496.

3

Transit Time Flow Measurement:

Principles and Clinical Applications

Jesper Laustsen, MD

Introduction

Intraoperative examinations of arterial, venous, or graft volume blood flow during vascular or cardiac surgery are necessary as quality control routines to document system behavior and to reveal technical errors. Several methods have been used: the electromagnetic flowmeter and ultrasound Doppler methods are now largely abandoned and have been replaced by ultrasound transit time flowmeters.

Principles

Transit Time Flowmetry

A transit time flow probe for measurement of volume blood flow consists of 2 small piezoelectric crystals, 1 upstream and 1 downstream, mounted in a common tip that can be clipped by a movable slider onto the vessel, without constriction. The front of the probe is flat, and a small metallic reflector bracket is mounted opposite the crystals. Each crystal can produce a wide ultrasound beam covering the entire vessel width. The

---

From: D'Ancona G, Karamanoukian HL, Ricci M, Salerno TA, Bergsland J (eds). *Intraoperative Graft Patency Verification in Cardiac and Vascular Surgery.* © Futura Publishing Company, Armonk, NY, 2001.

65

signals are visualized in real-time mode with relevant alphanumeric variables including absolute volume blood flow in mL/min.

The "transit times" are measured for an ultrasound pulse signal emitted from the upstream crystal to arrive at the downstream crystal via the reflector and for a signal from the downstream crystal to reach the upstream crystal via the reflector. Since ultrasound travels faster when it is transmitted in the same direction as flow, a small time difference for the 2 signals as expressed in a shift of phase (down to picosecond values) can be determined.

The angle between the probe and the vessel is not critical since upstream as well as downstream crystals are mounted in fixed positions within the probe. An increase of the angle between the upstream probe and the vessel will always be compensated by a corresponding decrease of the angle between the downstream probe and the vessel and vice versa.

All blood flow velocity components are detected by the wide ultrasound beam, and transit time determinations are sampled at all points across the vessel diameter, so the measurement of volume blood flow is theoretically independent of the blood flow velocity profile due to this integration procedure (Fig. 1).

The first transit time flowmeter was described by Franklin et al.[1] and Plass,[2] but the theoretical basis for volume flow measurements with the transit time principle was developed by Drost.[3]

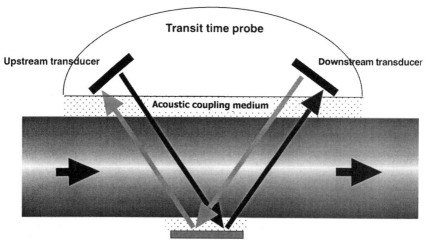

Figure 1. Schematic drawing of the transit time principle for measurement of volume blood flow. The arrows indicate the directions of the ultrasound beams and volume blood flow, respectively.

Transit time flowmetry is theoretically independent of internal or external vessel diameters, vessel shape, and blood flow profiles. It is, in contrast to ultrasound Doppler techniques, insensitive to the alignment between probe and vessel. The probe does not have to be in direct contact with the vessel wall, but acoustic fluid (gel, blood) must be present between blood vessel and probe to ensure good acoustic coupling. Homogeneous distribution of blood flow within the cross-sectional area of the vessel is not necessary. The volume flow measurement is independent on hematocrit fraction, on the value of the heart rate, and on the thickness of the vessel wall. There is no zero drift of the recorded signal, and calibration is unnecessary.

The flat probe design reduces the risk of trapping air between the probe and the vessel wall. In practice, the diameter of the probe should correspond well to the outer diameter of the vessel in order to obtain optimal acoustic contact.

Transit time technology has been shown to correlate well to esophageal ultrasound Doppler and to the thermodilution technique for measurement of cardiac output in pigs,[4] to thermodilution methods for pulmonary arterial and portal venous blood flows in pigs,[5] to direct (exsanguination) carotid artery flow determination in sheep and in vitro,[6] and to electromagnetic flowmeters in ascending aortas in dogs and abdominal aortas in cats.[7] In rats, 1- and 2-mm probes were used for measurements of mesenteric artery and aorta blood flows[8] where the 2-mm probe slightly overestimated flow in the medium range. An in vitro study showed a slight overestimation of blood flow with the transit time technique but showed excellent correlation between transit time and directly measured blood flow. Additional in vivo measurements on 9 saphenous vein grafts for aortocoronary bypass with transit time and ultrasound Doppler showed excellent agreement with a correlation coefficient of 0.990 at a transit time blood flow $=1.3 \pm 1.00 \cdot$ Doppler blood flow.[9]

During operations, volume blood flows were measured simultaneously by exsanguination from the cut distal end of the saphenous vein graft or the in situ internal thoracic artery and by the transit time flowmeter equipment. Within the examined blood flow range, the volume blood flow determined by the transit time method corresponded to the directly measured blood flow. For saphenous vein grafts and for in situ internal thoracic artery grafts, excellent correlation was demonstrated[10] (Fig. 2 a,b).

Clinical Applications

The features of the second generation transit time flowmeter differ from those of the first generation flowmeters by having real-time online

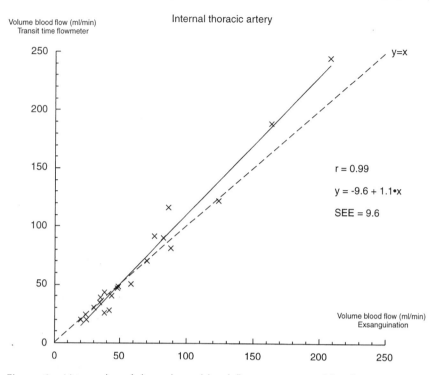

Figure 2a. Linear plot of the volume blood flow as measured by the transit time method (y) against volume blood flow as determined by exsanguination (x) during myocardial revascularization with the internal thoracic artery as coronary bypass (21 measurements in 12 patients). SEE is standard error of the estimate, and r is the correlation coefficient. The straight line was calculated by least squares regression analysis. The interrupted line represents y = x.

visualization of flow curves on a color monitor screen and by being built with memory for storage and post-processing.

Due to the air contents of polytetrafluoroethylene (PTFE) or coated Dacron grafts, transit time ultrasound cannot be used for measurements of flow in these grafts since air attenuates ultrasound.

The possibility to inspect real-time blood flow waveforms instead of ultrasound Doppler velocities is a major advantage of the transit time system, especially during papaverine tests after cardiovascular reconstructions.

The agreement between the transit time volume blood flow values and the directly measured blood flows has made the present technology the method of choice for routine clinical uses for measurement of volume blood flow in grafts and native vessels. At our institution, transit time flow measurement has been used successfully in arteries and veins in any

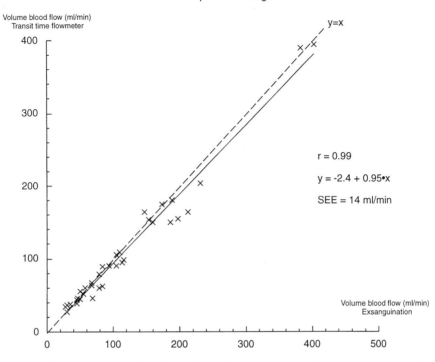

Figure 2b. Linear plot of the volume blood flow as measured by the transit time ul-trasound method (y) against volume blood flow as determined by exsanguination (x) during in situ saphenous vein grafting for critical leg ischemia (35 measurements in 13 patients). SEE is standard error of the estimate, and r is the correlation coefficient. The straight line was calculated by least squares regression analysis. The interrupted line represents y = x.

anatomical location whenever perioperative blood flow measurement is required.

References

1. Franklin DL, Baker DW, Rushmer RF. Pulsed ultrasonic transit time flowme-ter. IRE Transact Bio-Med Electronics 1962; 9:44–49.
2. Plass KG. A new ultrasonic flowmeter for intravascular application. IEEE Trans Bio-Med Eng 1964; BME-11:154–156.
3. Drost C. Vessel diameter-independent volume flow measurements using ul-trasound. Proc San Diego Biomed Symp 1978; 17:299–302.
4. Wong DH, Watson T, Gordon I, Wesley R, Tremper KK, et al. Comparison of changes in transit time ultrasound, esophageal Doppler, and thermodilution cardiac output after changes in preload, afterload, and contractility in pigs. Anesth Analg 1991; 72:584–588.

 5. Rubertsson S, Arvidsson D, Wiklund L, Haglund U. Comparison of blood flow measurement in the portal vein and pulmonary artery using transit-time ultrasound flowmetry and thermodilution techniques. Surg Res Comm 1993; 13:309–316.
 6. Lundell A, Bergqvist D, Mattson E, Nilsson B. Volume blood flow measurements with a transit time flowmeter: an in vivo and in vitro variability and validation study. Clin Physiol 1993; 13:547–557.
 7. Hartman JC, Olszanski DA, Hullinger TG, Brunden MN. In vivo validation of a transit-time ultrasonic volume flow meter. J Pharmacol Toxicol Methods 1994; 31:153–160.
 8. D'Almeida MS, Gaudin C, Lebrec D. Validation of 1- and 2-mm transit-time ultrasound flow probes on mesenteric artery and aortas of rats. Am J Physiol 1995; 268:H1368-H1372.
 9. Matre K, Birkeland S, Hessevik I, Segadal L. Comparison of transit-time and Doppler ultrasound methods for measurement of flow in aortocoronary bypass grafts during cardiac surgery. Thorac Cardiovasc Surg 1994; 42:170–174.
10. Laustsen J, Pedersen EM, Terp K, Steinbrüchel D, Kure HH, et al. Validation of a new transit time ultrasound flowmeter in man. Eur J Vasc Endovasc Surg 1996; 12:91–96.

4

Use of Transit Time Flow Measurement in Vascular and General Surgery

Anders Lundell, MD, PhD

Background and Technical Considerations

The success or failure of an arterial reconstruction is dependent on multiple factors: selection of patients, quality of inflow and outflow vessels, type of vascular conduit used, as well as surgical technique adopted. Several methods used for perioperative surveillance, such as angiography, angioscopy, continuous Doppler, and perioperative duplex, require expensive equipment, are highly dependent on the skill of the investigator, and have a considerable learning curve. In this context, an accurate measurement of blood flow would greatly enhance the information needed for the necessary perioperative evaluation of a peripheral vascular procedure. The method should be easy to use and present accurate and reproducible data. The primary aim of an intraoperative volume flow measurement is to obtain information on the immediate result of the reconstruction where a technical failure may jeopardize an otherwise successful operation. The measurement should give information on whether a revision is necessary. The measurement should therefore be made on the inflow and outflow vessels as well as the vascular conduit. Furthermore, it would be desirable to obtain information on both early and long-term prognosis of the reconstruction.

Flowmeter Methods

Invasive, quantitative flowmeters measure flow after placement of the flow probe directly on the vessel. These methods include the electromagnetic flowmeter, the Doppler flowmeter, and the transit time flowmeter (TTF).

From: D'Ancona G, Karamanoukian HL, Ricci M, Salerno TA, Bergsland J (eds). *Intraoperative Graft Patency Verification in Cardiac and Vascular Surgery.* © Futura Publishing Company, Armonk, NY, 2001.

Electromagnetic Flowmeter

Shercliffe described the theoretical basis of the electromagnetic flowmeter in 1962.[1] A bloodstream that flows at right angles through a magnetic field induces a voltage that is proportional to the flow velocity. Provided the cross-sectional area of the vessel is known, the flow is calculated automatically. The measurement is influenced by the hematocrit, the vessel wall thickness, as well as the angle between the probe and the vessel. The probe has to be calibrated before each measurement. The flow signal is unstable and the flowmeter has to be continuously recalibrated. These limitations may in part explain why this technology has never reached continuing widespread clinical use.

Doppler Flowmeter

The Doppler flowmeter was introduced in 1989. It requires no zeroing and measurements are virtually unaffected by the vessel wall. One transducer produces 2 pulsed Doppler ultrasonic beams.[2] The first is a wide beam that insonates the whole vessel area. The second is a narrow reference beam placed entirely within the bloodstream of the same cross-section to compensate for tissue attenuation. To minimize errors associated with angle insonation and vessel diameter, the transducer is fixed to the vessel wall at an angle of 50° with a special plastic cuff. The internal diameter of the vessel is measured manually. The flowmeter calculates volume flow from the measured mean velocity and vessel internal diameter.

Transit Time Flowmeter

In 1978 Drost et al. presented the theoretical basis for a flowmeter based on transit time ultrasound technique.[3] The transit time technique for measurement of flow has been known since 1969, but limitations in estimating vessel diameter and vessel misalignment, together with an unstable zero calibration, prevented its medical applications. These problems have been solved and the first self-calibrating TTF flowmeter was introduced in 1983. The TTF has been thoroughly validated.[4-7] It was immediately introduced in the experimental setting, and since the late 1980s has been used in in clinical settings. The introductory models, however, were based on an analog technology, making them somewhat sensitive to misalignment and kinking of the vessel. At sites of turbulence, there was a tendency for overestimation of flow leading to false high measurements. Digitalization of later models has compensated, to a certain extent, for those possible sources of error. The digital technology and the connection to a PC have also enabled online registration of flow as well as online calculation of resistance and impedance. The method is easy to use in a surgical setting during an operation and the presentation of data is stable and easily interpreted with only a short learning period.

The inadequacy of a TT flowmeter to measure flow in a newly inserted synthetic graft such as Dacron or PTFE is a drawback. This inability is, however, not unique for TT flowmeters. A similar problem was encountered with both the electromagnetic and the Doppler flowmeters. Caution must also be taken when the flow probe is placed in the immediate vicinity of a curvature or on a stenosed vessel. There is a tendency even with the modern digital TT flowmeters to overestimate flow in these situations. TTF could, however, be used as a completion control.

Femoropopliteal/Crural Reconstruction

Flow in femoropopliteal/crural bypasses has been investigated in a number of studies. Most of these studies are old and were done almost exclusively with electromagnetic flowmeters. Nonetheless, they showed a correlation between flow and patency. It seemed that a bypass flow of less than 70 mL/min at the time of surgery was an increased risk for graft thrombosis within the first postoperative months.[8–10]

The value of the measurement was furthermore enhanced by an intragraft injection of 30–40 mg of papaverine hydrochloride, which normally increases flow more than 100%.[11,12] An absence of flow increase could indicate a technical error or a compromised distal arterial bed. In spite of the fact that TTF has been available for clinical use for the last 10 years, there is to date no retrospective or prospective published study based on TTF of femoropopliteal/crural bypass flow and its correlation to patency.

Resistance

A further increase in prognostic value might be achieved when the measurement of flow is coupled to an intragraft measurement of pressure, thus making it possible to calculate peripheral resistance (mean arterial pressure/mean flow). TTF has been used to measure flow and calculate peripheral resistance in patients operated on for a femoropopliteal/crural bypass. Occluded bypasses have a median peripheral resistance of 1.24 compared to 0.63 in patent ones.[15] These numbers correlate closely to values obtained through other resistance measurement methods.[16–23] In this context, it must be pointed out, however, that not all authors agree that outflow resistance or flow predicts patency.[24]

Impedance

Further information can be obtained through impedance calculations. The digital TT flowmeters contain software that makes it possible to calculate impedance online.[25] Flow, resistance, and impedance are important factors in the outcome of an infrainguinal reconstruction. The inner diameter and the length of the conduit are probably just as important.[26]

Residual Arteriovenous Fistulae

Residual arteriovenous fistulae can be identified through a simple measurement of volume flow.[13] The flow probe is placed on the graft at the proximal anastomosis. The graft distal to the probe is digitally occluded. When no arteriovenous fistula is present between the occluded graft and the probe, graft flow is reduced to 0 mL/min. Graft flow only slightly decreases in the presence of an arteriovenous fistula between the compressed graft and the probe.[14]

Carotid Endarterectomy

TTF has been used for measurements of carotid artery flow both before and after carotid endarterectomy.[27–31] The need for completion control after carotid endarterectomy is apparent since early occlusion or embolization from the endarterectomy site may result in a perioperative stroke.[32,33] The risk of restenosis is increased if technical imperfections during the initial operation remain undetected. Impairments of flow could necessitate immediate reintervention before occlusion or embolization occur. The absolute values of blood flow vary considerably between individuals depending on severity of contralateral disease and established collaterals. Consequently, the relative alterations in flow seem to be more important than a defined volume flow. The lack of morphological information by transit time flowmetry is compensated by the gained functional information about the actual blood flow situation. Before the endarterectomy is performed, measurements show an overestimation of internal carotid artery stenosis.[34,35]

After the endarterectomy, there is a substantial redistribution of carotid artery blood flow.[36–40] The "overshoot" in blood flow after the operation could be due to a reactive hyperemia or to alterations in flow distribution due to autoregulative processes.[41]

Angioaccess

In the USA, vascular access thrombosis accounts for at least 1 billion dollars in annual expenses and 25% of hospitalizations for patients in chronic hemodialysis.[42] Low blood flow (between 300 and 800 mL/min) at the level of the vascular access modestly increases the relative risk for thrombosis in the short-term perspective.[43–45]

TTF can be used together with the ultrasound dilution technique to establish patency and to prognosticate function of angioaccess grafts and as a completion control after surgery.[46] The ultrasound dilution technique has even raised the possibility to monitor flow through PTFE access grafts.[47,48]

General Surgery

The use of TTF in general surgery is thus far devoted mainly to hepatic surgery. A number of studies have evaluated the interaction between hepatic arterial and portal venous flow, including the influence of positive end-expiratory pressure (PEEP) on hepatic blood flow and oxygenation. The collected TTF data indicate that a decrease in portal venous flow immediately gives rise to a significant increase in hepatic artery circulation. However, a decrease in hepatic arterial flow does not automatically lead to increased portal venous flow.[49] PEEP ventilation significantly decreased portal venous blood flow while hepatic blood flow was preserved by a compensatory increase in hepatic arterial blood flow. Mesenteric and hepatic oxygen delivery changed according to blood flow. Regulation of hepatic blood supply, not related to sympathetic activity, maintained liver oxygenation during PEEP ventilation despite a simultaneous decrease in mesenteric perfusion.[50,51] Ventilation with PEEP reduced CO and MAP levels and, as a consequence, decreased systemic and splanchnic oxygen; lactate concentrations, however, were unchanged.[52]

Conclusion

As a concluding remark regarding TTF in peripheral vascular surgery and general surgery, it can be stated that TTF flowmetry can be accomplished with reliable accuracy and reproducibility. It is important, how-ever, to stress that flow measurements do not replace other methods for perioperative surveillance in vascular and general surgery. The measure-ment of flow is merely another source for obtaining information. The prognostic value of the measurement should not be overestimated. It gives a momentary picture of bypass or angioaccess function albeit under simi-lar circumstances for each patient. In order to ascertain true prognostic value, flow recordings should be possible online over a prolonged post-operative period such as the first 24 hours after surgery.[53]

References

1. Shercliffe JA. The Theory of Electromagnetic Flow Measurement. Cambridge, Cambridge University Press, 1962.
2. Beard JD, Scott DJA, Evans JM, Skidmore R, Horrocks M. A Doppler flowme-ter for use in theatre. Ultrasound Med Biol 1986; 12:883–889.
3. Drost CJ. Vessel diameter independent volume flow measurements using ul-trasound. Proc San Diego Biomed Symp 1978; 17:299–302.
4. Mortensen FB, Rasmussen JS, Viborg O, Laurberg S, Pedersen EM. Validation of a new transit time ultrasound flowmeter for measuring blood flow in colonic mesenteric arteries. Eur J Surg 1998; 164:599–604.
5. Laustsen J, Pedersen EM, Terp K, Steinbruchel D, Kure HH, et al. Validation of a new transit time ultrasound flowmeter in man. Eur J Vasc Endovasc Surg 1996; 12:91–96.
6. Lundell A, Bergqvist D, Mattsson E, Nilsson B. Volume blood flow measure-ments with a transit time flowmeter: an in vivo and in vitro variability and val-idation study. Clin Physiol 1993; 13:547–557.
7. Albäck A, Mäkisalo H, Nordin A, Lepäntalo M. Validity and reproducibility of transit time flowmeter. Ann Chir Gynaecol 1996; 85(4):325–331.
8. Sonnenfeld T, Cronestrand R. Prognostic significance of intra-operative blood transfusions and flow measurements in reconstructive vascular surgery. Acta Chir Scand 1979; 145:305–311.
9. Sonnenfeld T, Cronestrand R. Factors determining outcome of reversed saphenous vein femoropopliteal bypass grafts. Br J Surg 1980; 67(9):642–648.
10. Bush HL Jr, Corey CA, Nabseth DC. Distal in situ saphenous vein grafts for limb salvage: increased operative blood flow and postoperative patency. Am J Surg 1983; 145(4):542–548.
11. Schwartz M, Batri G. The papaverine test for blood flow potential of the pro-funda femoris artery. Surg Gynecol Obstet 1981; 153(6):873–876.
12. Dedichen H. The papaverine test for blood flow potential of ileofemoral arter-ies. Acta Chir Scand 1976; 142(2):107–113.
13. Lundell A, Nyborg K. Do residual arteriovenous fistulae after in situ saphe-nous vein bypass influence patency? J Vasc Surg 1999; 30:99–106.
14. Plate G. Flow measurements in femoropopliteal reconstruction. Medi-Stim Clinical Cases, 1997, No. 2.
15. Lundell A, Bergqvist D. Prediction of early graft occlusion in femoropopliteal and femorodistal reconstruction by measurement of volume flow with a tran-sit time flowmeter and calculation of peripheral resistance. Eur J Vasc Surg 1993; 7(6):704–708.

16. Davies AH, Magee TR, Baird RN, Horrocks M. Intraoperative measurement of vascular graft resistance as a predictor of early outcome. Br J Surg 1993; 80(7):854–857.
17. Schwartz LB, Belkin M, Donaldson MC, Knox JB, Craig DM, et al. Validation of a new and specific intraoperative measurement of vein graft resistance. J Vasc Surg 1997; 25(6):1033–1041.
18. Ascer E, Veith FJ, White-Flores SA, Morin L, Gupta SK, et al. Intraoperative outflow resistance as a predictor of late patency of femoropopliteal and infrapopliteal arterial bypasses. J Vasc Surg 1987; 5(6):820–827.
19. Ascer E, Veith FJ, Morin L, White-Flores SA, Scher LA, et al. Quantitative assessment of outflow resistance in lower extremity arterial reconstructions. J Surg Res 1984; 37(1):8–15.
20. Vos GA, Rauwerda JA, van den Broek TA, Bakker FC. The correlation of perioperative outflow resistance measurements with patency in 109 infrainguinal arterial reconstructions. Eur J Vasc Surg 1989; 3(6):539–542.
21. Cooper GG, Austin C, Fitzsimmons E, Brannigan PD, Hood JM, et al. Outflow resistance and early occlusion of infrainguinal bypass grafts. Eur J Vasc Surg 1990; 4(3):279–283.
22. Miller J, Walsh JA, Foreman RK, Dupont PA, Luethke R, et al. Vascular outflow resistance and angiographic assessment of lower limb arterial reconstructive procedures. Aust NZ J Surg 1990; 60(4):275–281.
23. Parvin SD, Evans DH, Bell PR. Peripheral resistance measurement in the assessment of severe peripheral vascular disease. Br J Surg 1985; 72(9):751–753.
24. Wolfle KD, Bruijnen H, Morski A, Kugelmann U, Campbell P, et al. The importance of graft blood flow and peripheral outflow resistance for early patency in infrainguinal arterial reconstructions. VASA 1999; 28(1):34–41.
25. Schwartz LB, Purut CM, Craig DM, Smith PK, Moawad J, et al. Measurement of vascular input impedance in infrainguinal vein grafts. Ann Vasc Surg 1997; 11(1):35–43.
26. Meyerson SL, Moawad J, Loth F, Skelly CL, Bassiouny HS, et al. Effective hemodynamic diameter: an intrinsic property of vein grafts with predictive value for patency. J Vasc Surg 2000; 31(5):910–917.
27. Whyman MR, Naylor AR, Ruckley CV, Wildsmith JA. Extracranial carotid artery flow measurement during carotid endarterectomy using a Doppler ultrasonographic flowmeter. Br J Surg 1994; 81(4):532–535.
28. Benetos A, Simon A, Levenson J, Lagneau P, Bouthier J, et al. Pulsed Doppler: an evaluation of diameter, blood velocity and blood flow of the common carotid artery in patients with isolated unilateral stenosis of the internal carotid artery. Stroke 1985; 16(6):969–972.
29. Benetos A, Safar ME, Laurent S, Bouthier JD, Lagneau PL, et al. Common carotid blood flow in patients with hypertension and stenosis of the internal carotid artery. J Clin Hypertens 1986; 2(1):44–54.
30. Wiberg J, Nornes H. Effects of carotid endarterectomy on blood flow in the internal carotid artery. Acta Neurochir (Wien) 1983; 68(3–4):217–26.
31. Vanninen R, Koivisto K, Tulla H, Manninen H, Partanen K. Hemodynamic effects of carotid endarterectomy by magnetic resonance flow quantification. Stroke 1995; 26(1):84–89.
32. Gordon IL. Effects of stenosis on transit-time ultrasound measurements of blood flow. Ultrasound Med Biol 1995; 21(5):623–633.
33. Gordon IL, Stemmer EA, Williams RA, Arafi M, Wilson SE. Changes in internal carotid blood flow after carotid endarterectomy correlate with preoperative stenosis. Am J Surg 1994; 168(2):127–130.

34. van Everdingen KJ, van der Grond J, Kappelle LJ. Overestimation of a stenosis in the internal carotid artery by duplex sonography caused by an increase in volume flow. J Vasc Surg 1998; 27(3):479–485.
35. Archie JP Jr, Feldtman RW. Critical stenosis of the internal carotid artery. Surgery 1981; 89(1):67–72.
36. Gordon IL, Weil DJ, Williams RA, Wilson SE. Intraoperative measurement of Javid shunt flow with transit-time ultrasound. Ann Vasc Surg 1994; 8(6): 571–577.
37. Blankensteijn JD, van der Grond J, Mali WP, Eikelboom BC. Flow volume changes in the major cerebral arteries before and after carotid endarterectomy: an MR angiography study. Eur J Vasc Endovasc Surg 1997; 14(6):446–450.
38. Sillesen H. The haemodynamic value of external carotid artery collateral blood supply in carotid artery disease. Eur J Vasc Surg 1988; 2(5):309–313.
39. Magee TR, Davies AH, Baird RN, Horrocks M. Blood flow in the internal carotid artery and velocity in the middle cerebral artery during carotid endarterectomy. Cardiovasc Surg 1994; 2(1):37–40.
40. Whyman MR, Naylor AR, Ruckley CV, Wildsmith JA. Extracranial carotid artery flow measurement during carotid endarterectomy using a Doppler ultrasonographic flowmeter. Br J Surg 1994; 81(4):532–535.
41. Gordon IL, Stemmer EA, Wilson SE. Redistribution of blood flow after carotid endarterectomy. J Vasc Surg 1995; 22(4):349–358; discussion 358–360.
42. Neyra NR, Ikizler TA, May RE, Himmelfarb J, Schulman G, et al. Change in access blood flow over time predicts vascular access thrombosis. Kidney Int 1998; 54(5):1714–1719.
43. Wang E, Schneditz D, Nepomuceno C, Lavarias V, Martin K, et al. Predictive value of access blood flow in detecting access thrombosis. ASAIO J 1998; 44(5):M555–558.
44. May RE, Himmelfarb J, Yenicesu M, Knights S, Ikizler TA, et al. Predictive measures of vascular access thrombosis: a prospective study. Kidney Int 1997; 52(6):1656–1662.
45. Bosman PJ, Boereboom FT, Eikelboom BC, Koomans HA, Blankestijn PJ. Graft flow as a predictor of thrombosis in hemodialysis grafts. Kidney Int 1998; 54(5):1726–1730.
46. Depner TA, Krivitski NM. Clinical measurement of blood flow in hemodialysis access fistulae and grafts by ultrasound dilution. ASAIO J 1995; 41(3):M745–749.
47. Shackleton CR, Taylor DC, Buckley AR, Rowley VA, Cooperberg PL, et al. Predicting failure in polytetrafluoroethylene vascular access grafts for hemodialysis: a pilot study. Can J Surg 1987; 30(6):442–444.
48. Sands J, Glidden D, Miranda C. Hemodialysis access flow measurement: comparison of ultrasound dilution and duplex ultrasonography. ASAIO J 1996; 42(5):M899–901.
49. Jakab F, Rath Z, Schmal F, Nagy P, Faller J. The interaction between hepatic arterial and portal venous blood flows: simultaneous measurement by transit time ultrasonic volume flowmetry. Hepatogastroenterology 1995; 42(1):18–21.
50. Aneman A, Eisenhofer G, Fandriks L, Olbe L, Dalenback J, et al. Splanchnic circulation and regional sympathetic outflow during perioperative PEEP ventilation in humans. Br J Anaesth 1999; 82(6):838–842.
51. Doi R, Inoue K, Kogire M, Sumi S, Takaori K, et al. Simultaneous measurement of hepatic arterial and portal venous flows by transit time ultrasonic volume flowmetry. Surg Gynecol Obstet 1988; 167(1):65–69.

52. Berendes E, Lippert G, Loick HM, Brussel T. Effects of positive end-expiratory pressure ventilation on splanchnic oxygenation in humans. J Cardiothorac Vasc Anesth 1996; 10(5):598–602.
53. Cronestrand R, Ekestrom S. Blood flow after peripheral arterial reconstruction. I. Measurements after iliac-femoro-popliteal arterial reconstructions with the electromagnetic flowmeter and implanted flow probes during operation and in the early postoperative periods. Scand J Thorac Cardiovasc Surg 1970; 4(2):159–171.

5

Competitive Flow and Steal Phenomenon in Coronary Surgery

Giuseppe Speziale, MD

Introduction

The conventional strategy for coronary artery bypass grafting (CABG) includes use of left internal thoracic artery (ITA) and saphenous vein (SV) grafts.[1,2] In comparison with the SV, it has been shown that the left ITA has a better patency rate and leads to a superior event-free survival after 10 years.[3–7] These data encouraged use of bilateral ITAs and/or additional arterial conduits (i.e., gastroepiploic artery, inferior epigastric artery, radial artery) in order to achieve a total arterial myocardial revascularization.[8–10] The Y and T graft techniques have developed, with different free arterial conduits anastomosed off the side of an in situ ITA to reach different coronary segments.[11–13] When 3 or more arterial grafts are required, complete arterial grafting may be better achieved using sequential anastomotic or Y graft approach.[14,15]

Despite recent data that have confirmed better results of CABG when a complete myocardial revascularization is achieved using mainly arterial conduits, the Society of Thoracic Surgeons (STS) database reports a hospital mortality of 3.1%, a 1.4% incidence of sternal wound infection, a 4% rate of severe pulmonary dysfunction, a 6.4% rate of neurological events, and a 4% incidence of renal failure following CABG.[16,17] The mortality and morbidity rates increase, especially in high-risk patients including the elderly, patients with reoperations, and patients with left ventricular, pulmonary, and renal failure. The surgical access, together with the deleterious effects of cardiopulmonary bypass (CPB), and the possible neurological complications related to aortic manipulation play a

From: D'Ancona G, Karamanoukian HL, Ricci M, Salerno TA, Bergsland J (eds). *Intraoperative Graft Patency Verification in Cardiac and Vascular Surgery.* © Futura Publishing Company, Armonk, NY, 2001.

significant role in the mortality and morbidity rates. On this basis, coronary artery bypass surgery is actually focusing on less invasive surgical approaches, i.e., (1) off-pump coronary artery bypass (OPCAB), (2) port access, (3) minimally invasive direct coronary artery bypass (MID-CAB).[18–21]

The use of in situ and/or composite arterial grafts and the increasing popularity of less invasive CABG have raised interests and concerns about intraoperative evaluation of graft patency. Measurements of graft flow and coronary artery vascular resistance can be recommended after traditional CABG and/or after construction of composite arterial grafts performed under CPB conditions. They also should be considered mandatory after MIDCAB procedures. In this case, the left ITA harvesting can be achieved through a left anterior small thoracotomy, via a subxiphoid approach or thoracoscopically. When harvesting is made without thoracoscopy, the largest left ITA side branches cannot be divided and a controversy remains over the suspect intercostal steal phenomenon. Several studies investigated the impact of operative techniques and strategies on the long-term results of ITA grafting.

Variables analyzed include: relative patency of right ITA versus left ITA, free and/or composite grafts versus in situ left ITA, quality of target coronary vessels, degree of stenosis in the native coronary artery branches, harvesting techniques, single versus sequential grafting, use of Y or T techniques, and single versus bilateral ITA grafting.

In the last few years, competitive flow and steal phenomena have been hypothesized to be significantly correlated to the mechanism of graft failure. The competitive flow between native coronary arteries and grafts was considered a factor influencing early and late ITA patency rate.[22–32] In order to clarify this issue, we retrospectively analyzed patients who underwent CABG, including those receiving ITA to LAD grafting when a noncritical lesion of the native coronary artery was present.

A controversy exists about the possibility that undivided side branches may steal blood flow from the coronary circulation and lead to graft failure and angina.[33,34] However, many reports have demonstrated that the hemodynamic influence of patent left ITA muscular branches is poor, even in patients who underwent revascularization with composite arterial grafts.[35] In this case, some authors suggested the possibility of a diastolic steal phenomenon from one of the branches of the composite arterial grafts. Recently, we have investigated the hypothesis that a limited flow capacity of pedicled left ITA and/or competitive flow from one branch of the Y graft may result in insufficient flow to the revascularized coronary artery and produce diastolic steal.

Variables Influencing Early and Late Patency of Internal Thoracic Artery Grafts

Patency of the Internal Thoracic Artery Grafts

One of the initial indications for the use of the ITA was the presence of a recipient coronary artery of equal or smaller luminal size. The criterion has been revised after demonstrating that ITA grafts adapt to local blood flow demand.[4,5]

Recently, a wide variety of reports have documented excellent long-term patency rate of ITA grafts. The probability of a left ITA graft being patent at 10 years is 92% compared with 56% for an SV graft. In addition, the patency of an ITA free graft is similar to that of a pedicled graft.[3] The reasons for this are the anatomical and physiological characteristics of ITA conduits. ITAs are almost free from atherosclerosis and rarely develop intimal fibroplasia and/or atherosclerosis when used as bypass grafts. Several factors have been hypothesized to influence early and long-term patency of grafts (Table 1). Graft patency may be influenced by the patient's general status, by specific features of the graft (i.e., size, thickness of the wall, structure of the graft, length, incidence of spasm, and atherosclerosis), by the anatomy of the native coronary artery (i.e., site and severity of the stenosis, match between the graft and coronary artery), and by technical factors. (i.e., the surgeon's experience, harvesting technique).

The ITA grafts do not appear to be subject to the early thrombosis that occurs occasionally within vein grafts. When early ITA graft failure occurs, it seems to be related to subclavian occlusive disease, vasospasm, injury, or to an anastomotic imperfection. The normal ITA free flow from the cut end should be greater than 80 mL/min. A flow less than 40 mL/min

---

Table 1

Factors Influencing Early and Long-Term Graft Patency Rate

1. Technical Factors (the surgeon's experience)
   - extent of coronary artery disease (competitive flow)
   - choice of graft conduit
   - harvesting techniques (steal phenomenon)
   - anastomosis techniques

2. Patient-Related Factors
   - vasoregulatory response of conduit
   - endothelial characteristics of conduit
   - size match with native coronary artery
   - patient-related factors (age, gender, other noncoronary disease)

---

after pharmacological dilatation is considered inadequate and, in this case, the ITA is not suitable for coronary bypass grafting.

Competitive Flow Between ITA Grafts and Coronary Artery Branches

Native coronary arteries receive the highest blood perfusion during diastole with a significant decrease in early systole. Intraoperative flow measurements of ITA coronary artery bypass grafts may show a transition from a predominant systolic peak to a predominant diastolic peak. When the ITA is grafted to a severely stenotic coronary artery, the prevalent graft flow pattern is diastolic with a low systolic peak. On the other hand, the competitive flow between a moderately stenotic coronary artery and an ITA graft produces a flow pattern characterized by systolic reversal with a predominant diastolic peak. With the physiological delay of systolic pulse at the distal ITA, the left ventricular contraction reverses flow retrogradely into the ITA graft.

The coronary artery revascularized is one of the most important factors in determining the long-term patency of an ITA graft. The runoff of the coronary artery may contribute to late patency.[6] The ITA regulates its blood flow thanks to an autoregulatory response mediated by functioning vascular smooth muscle. Many authors demonstrated that the ITA responds to changes in flow demand due to the progression of stenosis in the native coronary artery.[22–24]

Although controversy exists, it has been hypothesized that competitive flow between the graft and the native coronary artery may produce late ITA graft failure[26,36,37] when the ITA is grafted to a coronary artery with a mild or moderate stenosis. In this setting, the ITA graft may gradually diminish in size (the so-called "string sign" or "distal thread sign") and graft failure may occur. The string sign refers to an angiographic typical picture of low or no flow through the in situ ITA graft. This phenomenon is difficult to predict because it is not constant, even when there is a consistent flow through the native coronary artery.[27] It was demonstrated that the ITA increases its diameter and flow when stenosis of the native coronary artery increases. The string sign is consequent to good native coronary flow and causes no clinical problems. In the absence of spasm, bypass conduit fibrosis, coronary runoff reduction, or harvesting injury, the angiographic signs of ITA narrowing may be considered as a physiological autoregulatory graft response to blood flow demands. However, although the string sign certainly occurs, it may be considered a dynamic and reversible phenomenon as demonstrated by Kitamura and associates.[25] In patients with a string sign of the ITA, temporary occlusion of the grafted coronary artery with a percutaneous transluminal coronary angioplasty balloon demonstrates anatomical patency of the ITA.[25] Thus, the reversible process that results in apparent graft occlusion supports the concept of "disuse atrophy" as proposed in 1974. The definition of atrophy is inappropriate because it refers to permanent changes. On the contrary, ITA grafts may continuously maintain anatomical patency even under no-flow situations just like nonfunctioning collateral vessels and may function properly later as a graft when the native coronary flow decreases.

To improve long-term CABG outcomes, quality of life, reduce angina, and reduce the reoperation rate, the surgical indications for CABG were extended to include patients with mild or moderate stenosis.[27] Results from experimental studies have demonstrated that competitive flow from a fully patent native coronary artery did not eliminate ITA graft flow. Kawasuji et al. analyzed patients in whom coronary arteries with less than 75% reduction in luminal diameter were occasionally bypassed when operation was indicated for a substantial lesion in another vessel.[28] The analysis of measurements of blood flow in ITA grafts demonstrated no significant difference of peak diastolic flow between groups of patients with different degrees of coronary stenosis. Angiography at 1 month demonstrated that ITA narrowing had developed in only 2 out of 13 ITAs grafted on a coronary artery with 50% stenosis or less. Thus, ITA grafting for coronary arteries with noncritical lesions did not cause an elevated incidence of string signs and it may be considered acceptable.

Spence et al.[38] reported that ITA graft flow is not influenced by the normal coronary vessel in a canine model and its flow is greater when attached in situ. The competitive flow may not be the cause of ITA narrowing and ITA graft flow depends on the flow required in the runoff bed and relative size of the native coronary arteries and graft.

A report by Urschel et al. suggested that competitive flow does not affect graft patency at 1 to 7 years follow-up.[39] Seki and associates[29] have demonstrated the quantitative relationship between the recipient coronary artery stenosis and graft diameter in postoperative angiographic evaluation. They considered the string sign to be benign if perioperative damage of the graft could be excluded. It is important to differentiate the anatomical occlusion derived from ITA injury (i.e., thermal, dissection, intramural hematoma, intimal fibrosis, severe pericardial inflammatory disease following CABG) from physiological occlusion. If the string signs are observed early after CABG, they may represent a technical error in harvesting and grafting.

Hashimoto et al.[30] showed that the degree of recipient coronary artery stenosis was the only significant predictor of graft patency. A more severe degree of stenosis (>60%) in the native coronary artery was present in patent grafts. It is clear that a number of studies will be necessary to clarify this issue. In particular, the concept of prophylactic grafting of noncritical lesions at the time of operation for another significant stenosis is the main challenge. Usually, the ITA is preferentially anastomosed to the most important coronary artery, the left anterior descending (LAD) artery, because of its excellent long-term patency rates. We consider that ITA grafting for mild or moderate LAD coronary artery stenosis may be acceptable. The trend toward a complete myocardial revascularization with arterial grafts and the use of prophylactic grafting of coronary arteries with noncritical lesions are still controversial.

Clinical Results

We have performed an angiographic follow-up in 122 patients who had undergone CABG 3 months to 10 years before. All patients had received left or right ITA on LAD and additional arterial and/or vein grafts to other coronary arteries. We included 11 patients with noncritical lesions on LAD who underwent ITA grafting with concomitant critical obstruction in other vessels. Patients received a total of 348 grafts. The mean number of arterial grafts was 1.6. All data were saved on a computerized database and reviewed by a cardiologist and a surgeon. A distal narrowing of the ITA grafting to a critically stenosed LAD was detected in 3 patients (2.4%). In these cases, early postoperative coronary angiography (3–6 months after surgery) was performed in response to symptoms suggestive of myocardial ischemia. Temporary occlusion of the native vessel did not restore blood flow through the ITA graft and an ITA injury during harvesting was suspected. A percutaneous transluminal angioplasty of the ITA grafts was performed showing excellent bypass flow. In all patients with noncritical lesions of the native coronary arteries, the ITA to LAD graft was patent despite evidence of a competitive flow (Figure 1).

Conclusion

In summary, it is thought that competitive flow between native coronary arteries and ITA graft flow may produce a distal ITA narrowing with development of string sign. The retrograde systolic flow and lower diastolic flow may influence endothelial signals and downsize distal ITA. Even in the presence of maximal competitive flow, the ITA graft flow is maintained and distal ITA narrowing has been demonstrated to be a reversible phenomenon whenever the native vessel is occluded. Thus, the ITA grafts may be considered dynamic conduits preserving their patency despite low-flow conditions. Conversely, the target vessels for the inferior epigastric artery and the right gastroepiploic artery must be those with

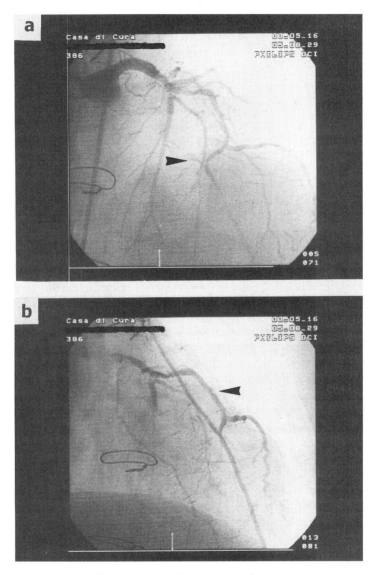

Figure 1. (a) Angiography at 10 years after CABG. Selective coronary angiography showing a noncritical lesion of the middle left anterior descending and systolic backflow through the distal internal thoracic artery graft (black arrow). (b) Selective injection of the internal thoracic artery showing graft patency with noncritical coronary artery stenosis (black arrow). (Reproduced with permission of Dr. Paolo Pantaleo.)

complete occlusion or severe stenosis and low coronary resistance. It is clear that a number of prospective studies will be necessary to clarify the relationship between string sign and:

• native coronary artery stenosis degree
• size match between graft and coronary artery
• runoff of the target coronary vessel
• endothelial signals
• patient-related factors.

Steal Phenomenon from Internal Thoracic Artery Side Branch

The ITA graft is considered the graft of choice for the LAD. To increase the number of arterial anastomoses per patient, both ITAs skeletonized, composite arterial graft with Y or T technique have been introduced. Because of the excellent long-term patency rate of ITA grafts, surgical techniques for complete arterial myocardial revascularization without the use of an SV graft were attempted.

Recently, there has been a great deal of investigation into the impact of operative techniques and strategies to improve long-term outcome of CABG.[19] In order to reduce morbidity or "invasiveness" of the procedure, the concept of minimally invasive has been introduced. When a single target vessel needs to be grafted, a MIDCAB procedure may be performed with limited access incision and avoiding CPB. During MIDCAB procedure, the ITA harvesting can be direct (or with video assistance), totally thoracoscopic, and via a subxiphoid approach.

However, only the thoracoscopic approach includes complete harvesting of the ITA with ligation of the intercostal side branches. This has been hypothesized to be a potential mechanism of coronary blood flow steal. Several studies reported resolution of angina after complete embolization of large ITA collateral branches and suggested dividing all ITA side branches.[33,34] Calafiore and associates demonstrated that the persistence of unligated side branches does not influence blood flow to the LAD artery after acute adenosine-induced myocardial hyperemia.[18,40] In fact, the described steal phenomenon does not occur primarily because muscular and coronary territories have different flow patterns occurring during different phases of the cardiac cycle. It was demonstrated that the ITA often originates together with other branches of the subclavian artery.[41] This common origin was found in many asymptomatic patients who underwent post-CABG angiography. Therefore, the persistence of undivided ITA branches is frequent after surgery and is independent from the harvesting technique used. In addition, many new branches with different sizes have been detected in different segments of ITA, even when a complete and direct dissection of ITA was performed. Thus, a theoretical flow steal would be present in many patients who underwent CABG.[42] The flow steal is possible only when a massive pharmacological muscular vasodilatation is induced. Fortunately, since this situation does not occur in a clinical setting, the potential for steal seems to be minimal. Diversion of blood flow to the side branches may be related to technical errors, poor runoff of the ITA graft, or mismatch between the distal ITA and coronary artery.[43,44] The transit time flow measurement is effective in promptly detecting technical errors after CABG even without CPB. This method provides specific information about the graft patency through the analyses of curves, mean flows, and pulsatility index values.[45]

In conclusion, if flow steal derived from undivided and/or neoformed ITA side branch were a reality, the long-term patency of CABG with use of ITA would not be so excellent. However, diversion of flow to muscular arteries may be frequently associated with graft failure due to stenotic anastomosis, poor runoff, and injury of the distal ITA. The technical factors influencing graft patency represent the true steal phenomenon. Intraoperative evaluation of graft status improves early and long-term results of CABG, reduces postoperative events, and redo procedures rate.

Diastolic Steal Phenomenon in Composite Arterial Grafts and Impact of Native Coronary Artery Flow

We usually prefer to use bilateral ITAs as in situ grafts to achieve total arterial revascularization. However, when the length of both ITAs does not allow all coronary sites to be reached, the right ITA may be divided at its origin and anastomosed to the left ITA (45° Y graft) before CPB is started.[11–13,46–49] Alternatively, when pedicled ITAs are used and an anastomosis site is difficult to reach, we use the right gastroepiploic artery, the inferior epigastric artery, or the radial artery in composite grafts with an ITA as inflow conduit (side branches or lengthening). When a graft is anastomosed to the aorta, the impact of native coronary flow on graft blood flow cannot be measured while the aorta is clamped. Royse et al. investigated the effects of competition between native coronary flow and composite arterial grafts constructed with the left ITA.[50] Construction of Y grafts (with right gastroepiploic artery, inferior epigastric artery, or radial artery) in a composite fashion with the left ITA significantly increases maximum potential flow before conduit occlusion. This is because the resistance of both conduits is lower than that of each conduit alone. After distal anastomoses completion, measurements of proximal left ITA flow without the presence of native coronary flow revealed a reduction of potential maximum flow. The latter is due to the coronary artery vascular resistances. When the aortic clamp is removed, the impact of native coronary artery flow produces a reduction of the proximal ITA flow. The reduction in graft flow is proportional to the runoff of the coronary vascular bed and the extent of myocardial infarction and coronary artery disease. However, the grafts' flow increases after weaning from CPB. A composite arterial graft has an excellent flow reserve, calculated by dividing the maximum potential flow by the flow after CPB interruption. The flow reserve is 1.9- to 2.3-fold greater than flow after CPB weaning.

The nominal graft flow of left ITA to LAD ranges from 33 to 45 mL/min measured with the transit time flowmeter. Therefore, the estimated flow reserve of isolated left ITA to LAD graft is approximately 3. The construction of a composite arterial graft produces a significant increase in the proximal ITA mean flow. The flow reserve of these grafts is 1.9 to 3.0 greater than mean flow after CPB interruption. Many arterial conduits may be used in association with the pedicled left ITA in Y graft. The radial artery is the larger vessel and produces the maximum potential flow reserve of the composite conduit (Table 2).

The hypothesis that the flow reserve of pedicled ITA may not provide sufficient blood flow for extended left ventricular revascularization was suspected. This is because the proximal ITA to the Y graft was considered the flow limiting of the conduit. This concept has been supported on the

Table 2
Flow Reserve in Composite Arterial Conduits with Left ITA

Free mean flow of left ITA (mL/min)	127 ± 21
Left ITA to LAD mean flow (mL/min)	51 ± 8
Flow reserve of left ITA	2.6
Free mean flow of all composite grafts with a pedicled left ITA (mL/min)	176 ± 39
Right ITA	188 ± 29
Radial artery	191 ± 36
Right gastroepiploic artery	157 ± 21
Inferior epigastric artery	149 ± 19
Conduit flow before aortic clamp release (mL/min)	105 ± 11
Right ITA	46 ± 9
Radial artery	55 ± 16
Right gastroepiploic artery	43 ± 8
Inferior epigastric artery	37 ± 6
Flow reserve of composite grafts	1.9
Proximal left ITA graft flow at 1 year follow-up (Color Doppler) (mL/min)	133 ± 23
Flow reserve of composite graft at 1 year	+22%

basis of the physiology of the coronary artery circulation. This latter may be considered mainly diastolic and terminal circulation. Recently, we demonstrated that the proximal ITA has the potential to support sufficient flow through a composite arterial graft. At intraoperative blood flow measurements, temporary interruption of flow in one branch of the Y graft did not significantly affect the ITA to LAD flow. On the other hand, the temporary occlusion of distal ITA did not produce flow changes in the other branch. The composite arterial graft flow maintains a mainly diastolic pattern with a minimal or limited systolic spike. In order to avoid influence of competitive flow from native coronary artery, we enrolled patients with critical stenosis and expected high runoff. Patients received a mean of 2.9 grafts/patient. The Y composite grafts had been constructed using the right ITA, right gastroepiploic artery, and inferior epigastric artery anastomosed to the side of the left ITA. The latter was sutured to the LAD, while the other branch was used to reach diagonal, obtuse marginal, posterolateral, and posterior descending territories of the right coronary artery. However, we prefer to revascularize the left and right coronary arteries separately. This allows dividing coronary territories with different vascular resistances, inflow patterns, runoff, and systolic restriction of flow due to ventricular mass.

Recently we included composite arterial Y graft with the use of the radial artery. Patients received single and sequential bypass grafts. Sequential anastomoses allow the most efficient use of arterial conduits by optimizing the number of distal anastomoses. Sequential grafting produced nonsignificant differences in flow reserve of the composite and left ITA to LAD graft when compared to single grafting. Using intraoperative graft flow measurement, we have demonstrated that the flow reserve of pedicled ITA allows for sequential grafting in composite grafting. At 1-year follow-up patients remained angina-free. Our findings are in contrast with the previous studies demonstrating that ITAs' flow reserve may not be as great as that provided by saphenous vein grafts and that patients may experience ischemia under stress.[41,43,51] However, intraoperative measurements of graft blood flow may be influenced by surgical trauma, ITA harvesting technique, cardioplegia, systemic temperature, aortic clamping, and CPB time.[52–55]

Arterial grafts used for coronary surgery are conductance arteries. The endothelium and the smooth muscle in the arterial grafts are features common to other arteries. Most studies have shown that endothelium-dependent relaxation is an important part of the endothelium-smooth muscle interaction.[56–60] This interaction may play a key role in determining superior long-term results for the arterial grafts. Emphasis on harvesting and anastomosing techniques will enhance long-term patency rate. In fact, when the endothelium is intact, the antiplatelet function of nitric oxide and the balance between vasoconstrictor and vasodilator factors maintain a continuous graft vasodilatation and avoid platelet attachment. Impairment in endothelial function derived from harvesting injury activates a coagulation cascade with thrombotic effects and development of atherosclerotic plaque. This situation causes early graft occlusion.

The flow reserve of composite grafts increases significantly after surgery. In our experience, an increase equal to 22% of flow reserve in the composite conduit occurred at 1-year follow-up. A combination of dynamic (blood flow measurements), functional (exercise stress test), and anatomical (angiography) procedures indicate excellent quality of life and patency rate at follow-up. These findings demonstrate that arterial grafts adjust blood flow if the endothelium is preserved.

Intraoperative flow measurements and postoperative angiographic follow-up are important methods to document the quality of surgical strategy. The transit time flow measurement (TTFM) was demonstrated to be superior in direct real-time detection of flow independent of vessel size and Doppler angle.[61,62] The TTFM allows for intraoperative detection of graft failure by evaluation of flow pattern, pulsatility index (PI), and flow value. The flow value is not a sufficient indicator of graft stenosis because it may be influenced by many factors in the early postoperative time. The PI value (obtained by dividing the difference between the maximal and minimal flow by the value of mean flow; range 1 to 5) is an excellent predictor of the quality of the anastomosis. A PI value higher than 5 indicates graft failure. A low mean graft flow with satisfactory flow pattern and low PI do not indicate a need for graft revision.[15,45,63–67]

Conclusion

ITA flow-through depends mainly on the resistance of the revascularized coronary artery and on the degree of competitive flow from the native coronary circulation. The graft flow is lightly influenced by the conduit flow capacity. Adequate flow regulation according to myocardial supply produces good early and long-term results in the composite arterial graft. The hypothetical phenomenon of hypoperfusion in composite arterial grafts does not correlate to diastolic steal from one of the branches of the Y graft. The ITA pedicle provides sufficient flow to revascularize the anterior and lateral walls of the left ventricle. The main challenges for early and long-term graft occlusion remain the technical factors. Surgical, endothelial, and CPB-related factors may influence graft flow. The use of arterial grafts has superior early and long-term results. The arterial grafts have superior long-term patency when the endothelial function is preserved.

References

1. Barner HB, Standeven JW, Reese J. Twelve-year experience with internal mammary artery for coronary artery bypass. J Thorac Cardiovasc Surg 1985; 90:668–675.
2. Lytle BW, Loop FD, Thurer RL, et al. Isolated left anterior descending coronary atherosclerosis: long-term comparison of internal mammary artery and venous autografts. Circulation 1980; 61:869–874.
3. Loop FD, Lytle BW, Cosgrove DM, et al. Influence of internal mammary artery graft on 10-year survival and other cardiac events. N Engl J Med 1986; 314:1–6.
4. Green GE. Technique of internal mammary coronary artery anastomosis. J Thorac Cardiovasc Surg 1979; 78:455–461.
5. Singh RN, Beg RA, Kay EB. Physiological adaptability: the secret of success of the internal mammary artery grafts. Ann Thorac Surg 1986; 41:247–250.
6. Chow MST, Sim E, Orszulak TA, et al. Patency of internal thoracic artery grafts: comparison of right versus left and importance of vessel grafted. Circulation 1994; 90:129–132.
7. Pick AW, Orszuak TA, Anderson BJ, et al. Single versus bilateral internal mammary artery grafts: 10-year outcome analysis. Ann Thorac Surg 1997; 64:599–605.
8. Tector AJ, Kress DC, Downey FX, et al. Complete revascularization with internal thoracic artery grafts. Semin Thorac Cardiovasc Surg 1996; 8:29–41.
9. Fiore AC, Naunheim KS, McBride LR, et al. Fifteen-year follow-up for double internal thoracic artery grafts. Eur J Cardiothorac Surg 1991; 5:248–252.
10. Angelini GD, Bryan AJ, West RR, et al. Coronary artery byass surgery: current practice in the United Kingdom. Thorax 1989; 44:721–724.
11. Grandjean JG, Voors AA, Boonstra PW, et al. Exclusive use of arterial grafts in coronary artery bypass operations for three vessel disease: use of both thoracic arteries and the gastroepiploic artery in 256 consecutive patients. J Thorac Cardiovasc Surg 1996; 112:935–942.
12. Tector AJ, Amundsen S, Schmahl TM, et al. Total arterial revascularization with T grafts. Ann Thorac Surg 1994; 57:33–39.
13. Calafiore AM, Di Gianmarco G, Luciani N, et al. Composite arterial conduits for a wider arterial myocardial revascularization. Ann Thorac Surg 1994; 58:185–190.
14. Calafiore AM. Use of the inferior epigastric artery for coronary revascularization: operative techniques. Cardiothorac Surg 1996; 1(2):147–159.
15. Speziale G, Ruvolo G, Coppola R, et al. Intraoperative flow measurements in composite Y arterial grafts. Eur J Cardiothorac Surg 2000; 17:505–508.
16. Edwards FH, Clark RE, Schwartz M. Coronary artery bypass grafting: the Society of Thoracic Surgeons National Database experience. Ann Thorac Surg 1994; 57:12–19.
17. Data analyses of the Society of Thoracic Surgeons National Cardiac Surgery Database, the Fifth Year. January 1996.
18. Calafiore A, DiGianmarco G, Teodori G, et al. Midterm results after minimally invasive coronary surgery (last operation). J Thorac Cardiovasc Surg 1998; 115:763–771.
19. Allen KB, Matheny RG, Robison RJ, et al. Minimally invasive versus conventional reoperative coronary artery bypass. Ann Thorac Surg 1997; 64:616–622.
20. Subramanian VA, Sani G, Benetti FJ, et al. Minimally invasive coronary byass surgery: a multi-center report of preliminary clinical experience. Circulation 1995; 92(suppl):I645.

21. Calafiore AM, Gallina S, Iacò A, et al. Minimally invasive mammary artery Doppler flow velocity evaluation in minimally invasive coronary operations. Ann Thorac Surg 1998; 66:1236–1241.
22. Dincer B, Barner HB. The "occluded" internal mammary artery graft: restoration of patency after apparent occlusion associated with progression of coronary disease. J Thorac Cardiovasc Surg 1983; 85:318–320.
23. Singh RN, Sosa JA. Internal mammary artery: a "live" conduit for coronary bypass. J Thorac Cardiovasc Surg 1984; 87:936–938.
24. Suma H. Internal thoracic artery and competitive flow. J Thorac Cardiovasc Surg 1991; 102:639–640.
25. Kitamura S, Kawachi K, Seki T, et al. Angiographic demonstration of no-flow anatomical patency of internal thoracic-coronary artery bypass grafts. Ann Thorac Surg 1992; 52:156–159.
26. Mills NL. Physiologic and technical aspects of internal mammary artery-coronary artery bypass grafts. In Cohn L (ed): Modern Technics in Surgery. Mt. Kisco, NY, Futura Publishing Co, 1982; 48:1–19.
27. Cosgrove DM, Loop FD, Saunders CL, et al. Should coronary arteries with less than fifty percent stenosis be bypassed? J Thorac Cardiovasc Surg 1981; 82:520–530.
28. Kawasuji M, Sakakibara N, Takemura H, et al. Is internal thoracic artery grafting suitable for a moderately stenotic coronary artery? J Thorac Cardiovasc Surg 1996; 253–259.
29. Seki T, Kitamura S, Kawachi K, et al. A quantitative study of postoperative luminal narrowing of the internal thoracic artery graft in coronary artery bypass surgery. J Thorac Cardiovasc Surg 1992; 104:1532–1538.
30. Hashimoto H, Isshiki T, Ikari Y, et al. Effects of competitive flow on arterial graft patency and diameter. J Thorac Cardiovasc Surg 1996; 111:399–407.
31. Lust RM, Zeri RS, Spence PA, et al. Effect of chronic native flow competition on internal thoracic artery grafts. Ann Thorac Surg 1994; 57:45–50.
32. Barron DJ, Livesey SA. Patency of an internal thoracic artery graft despite maximal competitive flow. Ann Thorac Surg 1995; 59:1556–1557.
33. Hartz RS, Heuser RR. Embolization of IMA side branch for post-CABG ischemia. Ann Thorac Surg 1997; 63:1765–1766.
34. Schmid C, Heublein B, Reichelt S, et al. Steal phenomenon caused by a parallel branch of the internal mammary artery. Ann Thorac Surg 1990; 50:463–464.
35. Cohn WE, Suen HC, Weintraub RM, et al. The H graft: an alternative approach for performing minimally invasive direct coronary artery bypass. J Thorac Cardiovasc Surg 1998; 115:148–151.
36. Geha AS, Baue AE. Early and late results of coronary revascularization with saphenous vein and internal mammary artery grafts. Am J Surg 1979; 137:456–463.
37. Suma H. Internal thoracic artery and competitive flow. J Thorac Cardiovasc Surg 1991; 102:639–640.
38. Spence PA, Lust RM, Zeri RS, et al. Competitive flow from a fully patent coronary artery does not limit acute mammary graft flow. Ann Thorac Surg 1992; 54:21–26.
39. Urschel HC, Razzuk MA, Miller E, et al. Operative transluminal balloon angioplasty. J Thorac Cardiovasc Surg 1990; 99:581–589.
40. Luise R, Teodori G, Di Gianmarco, et al. Persistence of mammary artery branches and blood supply to the left anterior descending artery. Ann Thorac Surg 1997; 63:1759–1764.

41. Hamby RI, Aintablian A, Wisoff BG, et al. Comparative study of the postoperative flow in the saphenous vein and internal mammary artery bypass grafts. Am Heart J 1977; 93:306–315.
42. Calafiore AM, Contini M, Iacò AL, et al. Angiographic anatomy of the grafted left internal mammary artery. Ann Thorac Surg 1999; 68:1636–1639.
43. Flemma RJ, Singh HM, Tector AJ, et al. Comparative hemodynamic properties of vein and mammary artery in coronary bypass operations. Ann Thorac Surg 1975; 20:619–627.
44. Pragliola C, Gaudino M, Bombardieri G, et al. Patent side branches do not affect coronary blood flow in internal thoracic artery-left anterior descending anastomosis: an experimental study. J Thorac Cardiovasc Surg 1999; 118: 66–70.
45. D'Ancona G, Karamanoukian HL, Schmid S, et al. Graft revision after transit time measurement in off-pump coronary artery bypass grafting. Eur J Cardiothorac Surg 2000; 17:287–293.
46. Lytle BW, Arnod JH, Loo FD, et al. Two internal thoracic arteries are better than one. Presented at AATS Meeting, Boston, May 3–6, 1998.
47. Carrel T, Horber P, Turina MI. Operation for two-vessel coronary artery disease: midterm results of bilateral ITA grafting versus unilateral ITA and saphenous vein grafting. Ann Thorac Surg 1996; 62:1289–1294.
48. Cameron A, Davis KB, Green G, et al. Coronary bypass surgery with internal thoracic artery grafts: effects on survival over a 15-year period. N Engl J Med 1996; 334:216–219.
49. Fiore AC, Naunheim KS, Dean P, et al. Results of internal thoracic artery grafting over 15 years: single versus double grafts. Ann Thorac Surg 1990; 49:202–209.
50. Royse AG, Royse CF, Groves K, et al. Blood flow in composite arterial grafts and effect of native coronary flow. Ann Thorac Surg 1999; 68:1619–1622.
51. McBride LR, Barner HB. The left internal mammary artery as a sequential graft to the left anterior descending system. J Thorac Cardiovasc Surg 1983; 86:703–705.
52. Menichetti A, Tritapepe L, Ruvolo G, et al. Changes in coagulation patterns, blood loss and blood use after cardiopulmonary bypass: aprotinin vs. tranexamic acid vs. epsilon aminocaproic acid. J Cardiovasc Surg (Torino) 1996; 37(4):401–407.
53. Speziale G, Ruvolo G, Marino B. A role for nitric oxide in the vasoplegic syndrome. J Cardiovasc Surg (Torino) 1996; 37(3):301–303.
54. Ruvolo G, Speziale G, Greco E, et al. Nitric oxide release during hypothermic versus normothermic cardiopulmonary bypass. Eur J Cardiothorac Surg 1995; 9:651–654.
55. Ruvolo G, Greco E, Speziale G, et al. Nitric oxide formation during cardiopulmonary bypass. Ann Thorac Surg 1994; 57:1055–1057.
56. Ferroni P, Speziale G, Ruvolo G, et al. Platelet activation and cytokine production during hypothermic cardiopulmonary bypass: a possible correlation? Thromb Haemost 1998; 80(1):58–64.
57. Dignan RJ, Yeh T, Dyke CM, et al. Reactivity of gastroepiploic and internal mammary arteries: relevance to coronary artery bypass grafting. J Thorac Cardiovasc Surg 1992; 103:116–122.
58. Ochiai M, Ohno M, Taguchi J, et al. Response of human gastroepiploic arteries to vasoactive substances: comparison with response of internal mammary arteries and saphenous veins. J Thorac Cardiovasc Surg 1992; 104:453–458.

59. Chardigny C, Jebara VA, Acar C, et al. Vasoreactivity of the radial artery: comparison with the internal mammary artery and gastroepiploic arteries with implications for coronary artery surgery. Circulation 1993; 88:115–127.
60. Mugge A, Barton MR, Cremer J, et al. Different vascular reactivity of human internal mammary and inferior epigastric arteries in vitro. Ann Thorac Surg 1993; 56:1085–1089.
61. Canver CC, Dame N. Ultrasonic assessment of internal thoracic artery graft flow in the revascularized heart. Ann Thorac Surg 1994; 58:135–138.
62. Canver CC, Cooler SD, Murray EL, et al. Clinical importance of measuring coronary graft flows in the revascularized heart: ultrasonic or electromagnetic? J Cardiovasc Surg 1997; 38:211–215.
63. Walpoth BH, Bosshard A, Genyk I, et al. Transit time flow measurement for detection of early graft failure during myocardial revascularization. Ann Thorac Surg 1998; 66:1097–1100.
64. Louagie YAG, Brockmann CE, Jamart J, et al. Pulsed Doppler intraoperative flow assessment and midterm coronary graft patency. Ann Thorac Surg 1998; 66:1282–1288.
65. Walpoth BH, Muller MF, Genyk I, et al. Evaluation of coronary bypass flow with color-Doppler and magnetic resonance imaging techniques: comparison with intraoperative flow measurements. Eur J Cardiothorac Surg 1999; 15:795–802.
66. Pagni S, Storey J, Ballen J, et al. ITA versus SVG: a comparison of instantaneous pressure and flow dynamics during competitive flow. Eur J Cardiothorac Surg 1997; 11:1086–1092.
67. Barner HB. Blood flow in the internal mammary artery. Am Heart J 1973; 86:570–571.

6

Transit Time Flow Measurement in Off-Pump Coronary Artery Bypass Grafting:

The Buffalo Experience

Giuseppe D'Ancona, MD,
Hratch L. Karamanoukian, MD, Marco Ricci, MD,
Tomas A. Salerno, MD, Jacob Bergsland, MD

Introduction

The increasing popularity of coronary artery bypass grafting (CABG) performed on a beating heart without cardiopulmonary bypass (CPB) has raised interests and concerns about the quality of the anastomoses performed during these procedures. To prove the feasibility of off-pump CABG (OPCAB), intraoperative evaluation of graft patency has become essential. In the past, a wide variety of flow measurement techniques have been used to intraoperatively assess the quality of the anastomoses after traditional CABG performed under CPB conditions.[1,2] None of them, for many different reasons, has been properly applied clinically.

Transit time flow measurement (TTFM) has recently been introduced as an effective and reliable means for intraoperative evaluation of coronary grafts. This technology allows for flow determination independent of vessel size, shape, and Doppler angle used.[3] Exact interpretation of transit

From: D'Ancona G, Karamanoukian HL, Ricci M, Salerno TA, Bergsland J (eds). *Intraoperative Graft Patency Verification in Cardiac and Vascular Surgery.* © Futura Publishing Company, Armonk, NY, 2001.

time flow patterns is essential to correctly use this technology in both OP-CAB and traditional CABG.[4,5]

The objective of this chapter is to assess the clinical function of TTFM in detecting anastomotic imperfections following OPCAB. Our experience at the Center for Less Invasive Cardiac Surgery in Buffalo, New York, will be summarized, trying to define some guidelines for a correct interpretation of the intraoperative TTFM findings.

The Buffalo Experience

Materials and Patients

Since we started to perform OPCAB in 1995, many changes have been introduced to ameliorate the surgical conditions and to ensure a perfect quality of the anastomoses. Since March 1996, we have adopted different methods of intraoperative graft patency verification including electromagnetic, Doppler, and finally TTFM technologies. Initially, measurements were performed without a specific protocol and data were not stored for adequate analyses. Since May 1997, a research protocol has been started for intraoperative recording of TTFM findings in all patients operated without CPB. From May 1997 to December 1998, TTFM was evaluated in 409 patients undergoing OPCAB via median sternotomy. A total of 1145 grafts were tested with TTFM. Preoperative, intraoperative, and perioperative data were recorded for every patient. Information concerning the intraoperative flow characteristics, size, and quality of the revascularized vessels was recorded for every single anastomosis performed.

Surgical Technique

A standard surgical technique was used in all patients. After median sternotomy and conduit harvesting, the pericardium was opened and pericardial stay sutures were placed. Exposure of the different coronary branches was obtained placing the "single" suture in the oblique sinus of the pericardium.[6] Coronary stabilization was achieved with the CTS stabilizer (CTS, Cupertino, CA). Systematical proximal snaring (4–0 pledgetted suture) and intracoronary shunting of the involved coronary artery branches were used.

The distal anastomoses were performed with 7–0 Prolene® running suture. The proximal anastomoses were performed with 6–0 running Prolene suture on a partially excluded ascending aorta.

TTFM Principle

At the end of every single anastomosis, flow values and flow curves were obtained using the TTFM device (Medi-Stim BF 2004, Medi-Stim, Oslo, Norway). TTFM is a new ultrasound based technology. Ultrasounds are mechanical waves that, whenever traveling through biological tissues, produce different effects. The Doppler effect is at the base of the Doppler flowmetry, widely adopted in cardiac and vascular surgery. The transit time effect of ultrasound waves is at the base of TTFM. In summary, ultrasound waves that travel upstream in a vascular conduit will take a longer time than waves moving downstream. In a typical TTFM probe, 2 piezoelectric ultrasound crystals are placed on the same side of the probe. The distance and the angle between the 2 crystals are stable. The crystals are able to produce ultrasound waves whenever electrically stimulated and to produce "electrical signals" whenever hit by ultrasound waves. A metal reflector is placed on the opposite side of the probe (and consequently of the vessel). The distance and angle between these 3 parts of the TTFM probe are stable (Fig. 1). Every ultrasound signal produced is reflected by the reflector and passes twice through the blood vessel. The transit time is the time spent by an ultrasound signal to travel from one crystal to the other after being reflected by the reflector. A different transit time will be recorded if the ultrasound waves travel upstream (increased time) or downstream (reduced time). A highly sensitive device will measure the very small differences in transit time. The volume blood flow will be directly derived (the higher the transit time difference, the higher the blood flow).

TTFM Interpretation

During our clinical experience we developed progressive expertise in TTFM findings interpretation. Our personnel was trained by the manufacturing company and worked in close relationship with the surgical staff to properly interpret and store the TTFM findings. Specific rules were developed to correctly address the different TTFM findings including flow curves, pulsatility index (PI), and mean flow values (Fig. 2).

Flow Curve: The curves should always be coupled with the ECG tracing to correctly differentiate the systolic from the diastolic flow (Fig. 3). In a patent coronary graft, the hemodynamics are similar to those physiologically observed in the coronary circulation: blood flows mainly during diastole with minimal systolic peaks taking place during the isovolumet-

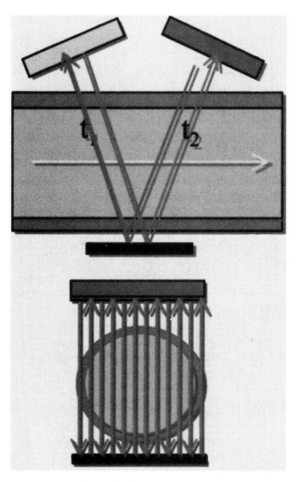

Figure 1. The TTFM principle: wide ultrasound beams travel upstream and down-stream. The difference in transit time (TT) is measured and is proportional to blood volume flow.

ric ventricular contraction (QRS complex) (Fig. 3). The diastolic filling pattern, typical of patent grafts, represents the antegrade flow that during every cardiac cycle flows from the graft to the coronary artery via the anastomosis. In contrast, the systolic peaks are not indicators of flow through the anastomosis and represent retrograde blood flow from the coronary artery into the graft. In this situation, during every systole, the blood is actively "squeezed" to flow backward into the graft (Fig. 3). Ideally, small systolic peaks should be found during intraoperative TTFM recordings. The curves are generally very similar when left anterior descending (LAD) or left circumflex grafts are tested (Figs. 4, 5). The right coronary artery (RCA) presents a particular flow pattern characterized

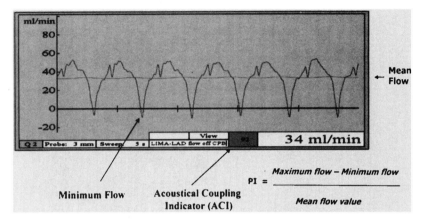

Figure 2. The TTFM curve parameters.

by a dual beat filling (Fig. 6). Flow in the right system is physiologically taking place during both phases of the cardiac cycle. As a result, patent grafts to the RCA may have TTFM curves with positive systolic peaks representing blood flow going antegradely from the graft into the coronary artery.

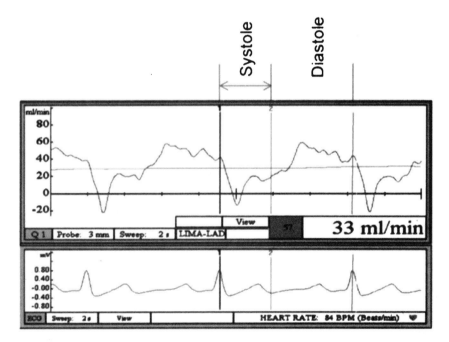

Figure 3. The TTFM curve should always be coupled with the ECG tracing to differentiate the systolic from the diastolic components of the flow.

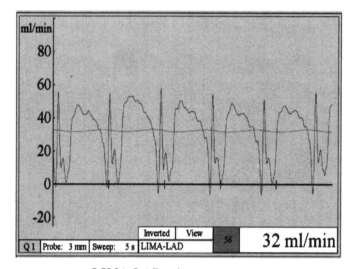

LIMA-LAD w/snare

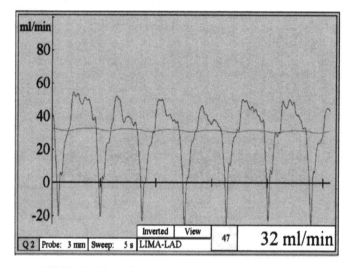

LIMA-LAD wo/snare

Figure 4. TTFM flow curve in a patent LIMA-LAD graft.

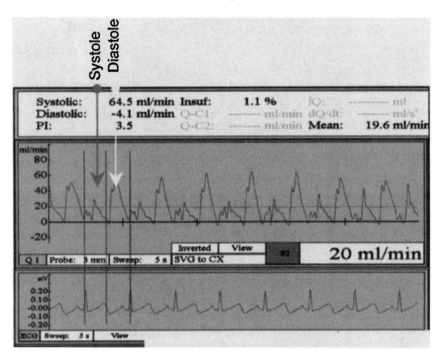

Figure 5. TTFM curve in a patent SV-CX graft.

Pulsatility Index: The PI, expressed as an absolute number, is a good indicator of the flow pattern and, consequently, of the quality of the anastomosis. This number is obtained by dividing the difference between the maximum and the minimum flow by the value of the mean flow (Max Flow − Min Flow/Mean Flow). In our experience, the PI should range from 1 to 5. The possibility of a technical error in the anastomosis increases for higher PI values.

Mean Flow: The mean flow is expressed in mL/min and, per se, is a poor indicator of the quality of the anastomosis. Too many variables are involved in determining the actual flow value and most of them are independent of the quality of the anastomosis. Flow (Q) is directly proportional to the perfusion pressure (P) and inversely proportional to the vascular resistance (R) as summarized by the first ohm law $Q = \Delta P/R$. R is inversely proportional to the fourth power of the vessel's radius, directly proportional to the length of the conduit in which the blood flows, and to the blood viscosity ($R = 8\eta\, L/\eta\, R4$, where η = viscosity, L = conduit length, R = conduit radius). Consequently, R is extremely elevated whenever the size of the revascularized vessel is reduced. This can cause

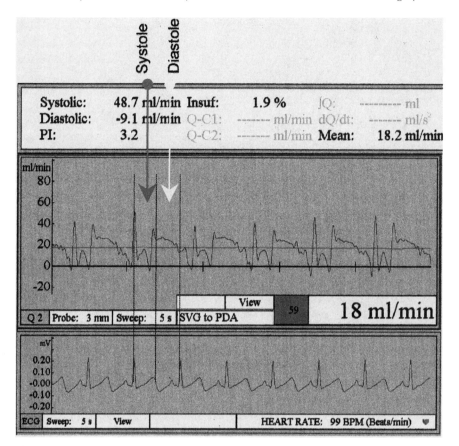

Figure 6. TTFM curve in a patent SV-RCA graft: note the "dual beat filling" pattern with positive systolic flow typical of the RCA grafts.

a drastic reduction in the actual flow value independent of the technical quality of the anastomosis. On the contrary, technically imperfect anastomoses may present with an "adequate" actual flow value if the size of the revascularized vessels is large and, as a consequence, the R tends to be lower.

TTFM Technique

The TTFM probe was perfectly fitted around the graft. Different probe sizes were available to avoid distortion or compression of the graft and to maximize contact between the conduit and the probe. Skeletonization of a small segment of the mammary artery was necessary to reduce the quantity of tissue interposed between the vessel and the probe. Aqueous gel was used to improve probe contact.

Flow measurements were routinely performed with and without proximal snare to evaluate patency of the anastomotic toe and heel (Fig. 7). The proximal and distal parts of the anastomosis were tested, in this way, excluding any possible form of competition from the native vessel (Fig. 7). Adequate de-airing of the grafts was performed, adequate systemic blood pressure was maintained, traction on the pericardium was released, and the stabilizer was removed from the epicardial surface to allow for the heart to return to its anatomical position. TTFM was repeated before chest closure to confirm graft patency and to detect any possible graft kinking or compression.

Results

Forty-one grafts (41/1145) were revised in 33 patients. In 3 patients, 4 flow curves and flow values were not properly stored in the TTFM device hardware and for this reason have not been included in this study.

A total of 37 grafts are included: 18 to the LAD and diagonal branches, 10 to the circumflex system, and 9 to the right coronary artery system (RCA) (Table 1). A total of 6 patients (18.1%) underwent graft revision on CPB. TTFM findings before revision are summarized in Table 1. Curve patterns, flow, and PI values remained unchanged after topical use of vasodilators (papaverine and nitrates).

Twenty-nine grafts (78.37%) were revised for abnormal (systolic) flow patterns, high PIs, and low flow values. In 5 cases (13.51%), despite abnormal flow curves (systolic spikes) and high PIs, flow values were on average greater than 15 mL/min. Findings at revision of these 34 grafts included: thrombosis of the anastomosis (6 patients), intimal flap or dissection in the native coronary artery (Figs. 8, 9) (5 patients), dissection of the internal mammary artery (5 patients), graft kinking (Figs. 10, 11) (4 patients), flap at proximal anastomosis (1 patient), stenosis at the toe or heel of the anastomosis (Fig. 12) (8 patients), coronary stenosis distal to the graft (Fig. 13) (3 patients), and no findings (2 patients). After revision, all flow patterns improved (diastolic flows) and mean flow values increased from a mean value of 3.85 ± 4.63 to 32.47 ± 28.59 mL/min with proximal snare ($P<0.0001$) and from 6.58 ± 6.00 to 36.29 ± 26.91 without snare ($P<0.0001$). PI values also improved from 38.45 ± 56.56 to 3.03 ± 1.6 with snare and from 24.44 ± 46.51 to 2.80 ± 1.68 without snare ($P<0.05$). TTFM findings after revision are summarized in Table 2.

In 3 additional grafts (8.1%), revision was performed on the basis of low mean flow values (mean 7.3 ± 2.51 mL/min with snare and 6 ± 1

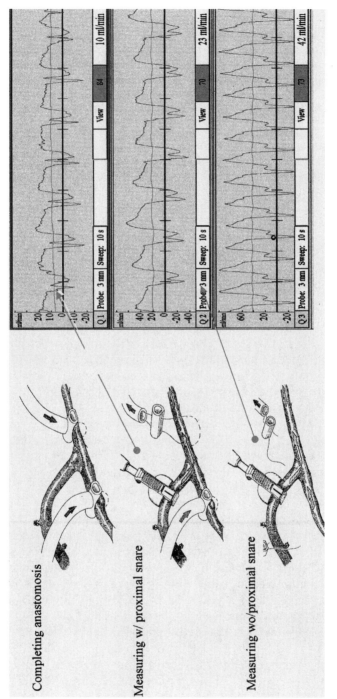

Figure 7. Snaring technique for TTFM.

Table 1
TTFM Findings in 37 Grafts before Revision

Type of Graft	% Coronary Stenoses	Size of Coronary (mm)	Mean Flow W/Wo Snare mL/min	PI W/Wo Snare	Resistance Ω W/Wo Snare	Flow Pattern
LIMA⇒LAD	90	2.5	0–1/0	60/60	78/78	Systolic
SVG⇒RCA	90	1.5	12/12	49/49	7.08/7.08	Systolic
LIMA⇒LAD	100	2	5/5	6.6/6	12/12	Systolic
SVG⇒RCA	70	2.5	3/3	55/50	25.6/25.6	Systolic
SVG⇒D	85	2.0	6/12	10.8/4.2	9/7.83	Systolic
LIMA⇒LAD	90	2.5	0/1	7/7	60/60	Systolic
SVG⇒RCA	**100**	**1.5**	**5/5**	**0/3.3**	**11/11**	**Diastolic**
LIMA⇒LAD	85	2	0/4	4.2/3.2	80/23.24	Systolic
LIMA⇒LAD	90	2.5	8/19	4.5/1	10.25/4.31	Systolic
LIMA⇒D	90	2	12/7	3/3	6.5/11.42	Systolic
RIMA⇒RCA	100	2.5	0/15	48/4.3	62/3.86	Systolic
SVG⇒CX	50	1.5	0/1	12.7/12.6	51/51	Systolic
SVG⇒OM	90	2.0	0/0	45.7/45.7	83/83	Systolic
LIMA⇒LAD	90	1.5	1/1	34.6/34.6	87/87	Systolic
SVG ⇒CX	90	1.5	0/0	22.1/22.1	67/67	Systolic
LIMA⇒LAD	**85**	**1.5**	**10/6**	**4.3/4.6**	**9.3/13.5**	**Diastolic**
SVG⇒RCA	80	2.0	0/14	10.4/2	73/5.7	Systolic
LIMA⇒LAD	90	2.0	1/4	14/4.9	69/17.5	Systolic
SVG⇒RCA	95	2.0	13/13	8.2/8.2	7.3/7.3	Systolic
LIMA⇒LAD	100	1.5	6/12	5.8/3.5	11.83/6.16	Systolic
LIMA⇒LAD	80	2.0	6/5	10/10	68/70	Systolic
SVG⇒OM	80	2.5	3/1	13.9/22	21.5/71	Systolic
SVG⇒OM2	90	2	0/10	225/6.5	70/7	Systolic
SVG⇒RCA	100	1.0	3/5	12/12	25.3/15.2	Systolic
SVG ⇒D	90	1.5	0/0	52.8/52.8	67/67	Systolic
SVG ⇒OM2	100	2.5	6/6	11.7/11.7	9/9	Systolic
SVG⇒LAD	90	1.5	0/11	58.4/2	86/8.3	Systolic
LIMA⇒LAD	**50**	**1.5**	**7/7**	**1.3/1.3**	**16.57/16.57**	**Diastolic**
LIMA⇒LAD	90	2.0	2/13	30.9/4.3	34/5.38	Systolic
SVG ⇒LAD	60	1.5	0/0	265/265	89/89	Systolic
SVG⇒CX	60	1.5	1/1	67.1/67.1	57/57	Systolic
SVG⇒RCA	70	2.0	11/11	10/10	60/60	Systolic
SVG⇒OM1	75	2.0	9/12	33.5/5	6.5/4.9	Systolic
SVG⇒D	75	2.0	0/0	70.5/11	74/74	Systolic
SVG⇒RCA	95	2.5	8/4	14/14	8/16.25	Systolic
SVG⇒OM2	100	1.5	0/2	16/10	100/50	Systolic
SVG⇒OM2	90	2.5	15/20	15/6.5	5.3/4.5	Systolic

Bold characters indicate grafts revised on the basis of low flow values despite normal flow patterns. Underlined characters indicate grafts revised on the basis of abnormal flow patterns despite flow values greater than 15 mL/min on average.
LIMA = left internal mammary artery; SVG = saphenous vein graft; RIMA = right internal mammary artery; LAD = left anterior descending; D = diagonal; RCA = right coronary artery; CX = circumflex coronary artery; OM = obtuse marginal.

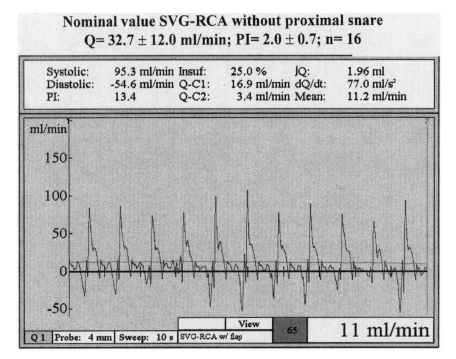

Figure 8. TTFM curve in a SV-RCA graft: note that in spite of a mean flow value of 11 cc/min, the flow curve appears to be "spiky" with mainly systolic flow and high PI values.

mL/min without snare) despite normal flow curves (diastolic) and PI values (1.86 ± 2.20 with and 3.06 ± 1.66 without snare). There were no findings at revision and curves, flow, and PI values remained unchanged after revision (Tables 1, 2).

Postoperatively, 1 patient developed a stroke (3%), 1 had an acute myocardial infarction (AMI) (3%), 1 required reoperation for bleeding (3%), 1 had a sternal wound infection, and 1 required prolonged ventilatory support (3%). All patients were discharged after a mean hospital stay of 8.15 days.

Discussion

CABG is a routine operation performed yearly on several hundred thousand patients. Although technical errors are possible during construction of coronary anastomoses, most of the time grafts are assumed to be patent, especially if constructed in a bloodless, motionless field as during cardioplegic arrest.

The recent popularity of OPCAB has revived interests and concerns about coronary graft patency. Although angiography remains the gold standard method to gain anatomical information about coronary grafts, its invasiveness and its lack of information about the functional status of the coronary anastomosis have confirmed the necessity to validate a less in-

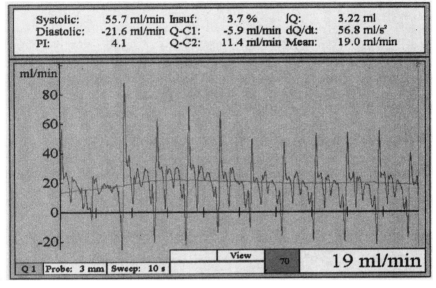

A

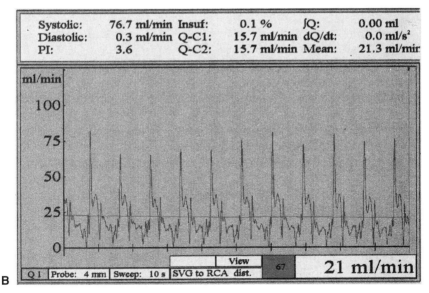

B

Figure 9. Flow curve after revision of the SVG to the RCA: at surgical revision, an intimal flap of the RCA was found.

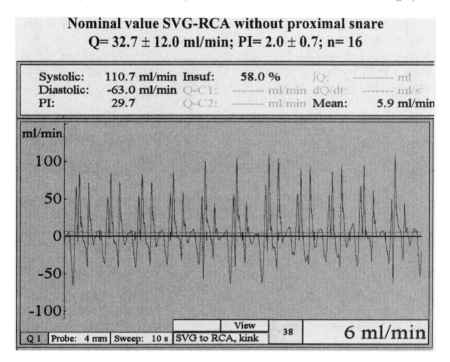

Figure 10. Abnormal TTFM curve in kinked SVG to the RCA: note the "spiky" shape of the curve with mainly systolic flow.

vasive and reliable method of intraoperative graft patency verification. In this regard, several techniques have been used in the past to intraoperatively test coronary graft flow.

Electromagnetic flowmeters, initially adopted in coronary surgery, have been recently replaced by ultrasonic technology (Doppler and TTFM). Many authors have demonstrated the superiority of TTFM over Doppler systems in direct real-time detection of blood flow.[2,3] Despite the tremendous improvements offered by the modern technology, many surgeons are still skeptical and misinformed about the applicability of modern flowmetry, and the vast majority of them[7] still use manual palpation as the preferred method to test graft patency after CABG. Most of the actual skepticism about intraoperative graft patency verification is also due to the failure that electromagnetic technology has had in the last decade. Electromagnetic devices measure the intensity of the electromagnetic field generated by the electrically charged red cells (iron bound to hemoglobin) that flow within the vessel. Actual blood flow is directly proportional to the intensity of the electromagnetic field generated. Many limitations have reduced the applicability of electromagnetic flowmetry. Ultrasound-based systems, and especially TTFM, offer many advantages and are more reliable for intraoperative verification of coronary graft patency. TTFM is theoretically independent of internal or external vessel diameter, vessel shape, and Doppler angle.[2,3] TTFM is also insensitive to the alignment between probe and vessel. The probe does not have to be in direct contact with the vessel, and zero calibration is not necessary. The recordings are stable and data storage and analysis are routinely done. Many of these features are not offered by Doppler technology.[2,3]

The TTFM device is very easy to use and requires no more than 30 seconds per measurement. Flow probe size varies from 2 mm to 32 mm and the most frequently used in cardiac surgery ranges between 2 mm and 3.5 mm. The probe is connected to a computer that has more than 200 MB memory and is programmed with software in Microsoft Windows format. Measurements are not influenced by the angle between vessel and probe, the hematocrit level, the heart rate, or the thickness of the vessel wall.

We began using TTFM routinely in off-CPB coronary surgery in 1996.[8] After 4 years of clinical experience, we believe that this technology

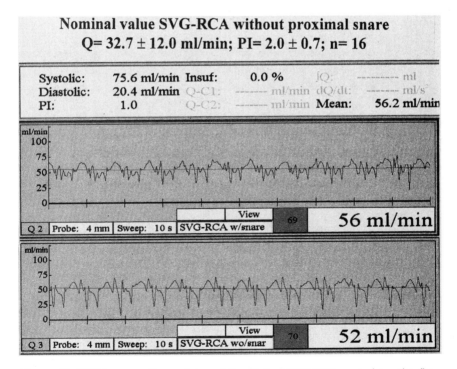

Figure 11. TTFM curve after revision of the kinked SVG-RCA: note how the flow curve is now mainly diastolic, the absolute flow value is increased, and the PI is reduced.

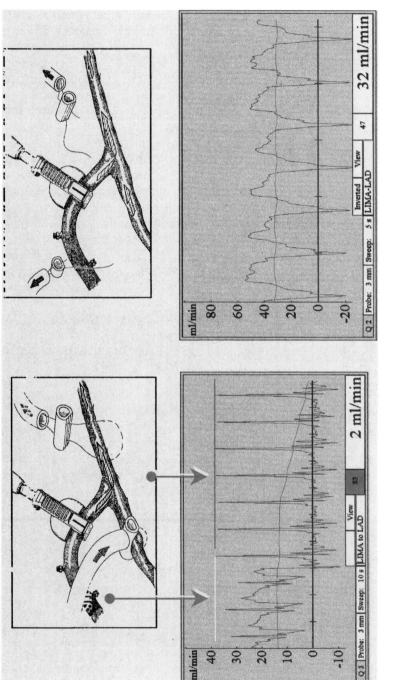

Figure 12. Abnormal TTFM curve of LIMA-LAD: note how the curve changes when the proximal snare is applied. At surgical revision, a significant stenosis was found on the native coronary distal to the site of the anastomosis.

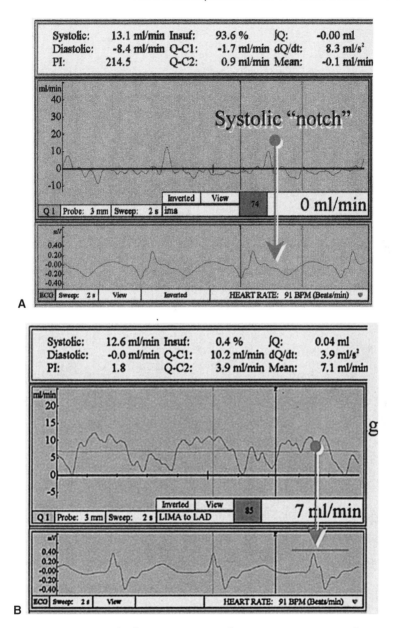

Figure 13. LIMA-LAD: in the first measurement the curve presents a systolic pattern with no flow and high PI values. At surgical revision a technical imperfection was found at the toe of the anastomosis. The TTFM curve is improved after revision (mainly diastolic flow) although the absolute flow remains low (probably due to poor runoff in the LAD territory).

Table 2
TTM Findings in 37 Grafts after Revision

Type of Graft	% Coronary Stenoses	Size of Coronary (mm)	Mean Flow W/Wo Snare mL/min	PI W/Wo Snare	Resistance Ω W/Wo Snare	Flow Pattern
LIMA⇒LAD	90	2.5	40/33	2/2.3	2/2.4	Diastolic
SVG⇒RCA	90	1.5	25/25	3/3	4/4	Diastolic
LIMA⇒LAD	100	2	41/41	1.5/1.5	1.41/1.41	Diastolic
SVG⇒RCA	70	2.5	10/10	8.7/8.7	10/10	Diastolic
SVG⇒D	85	2.0	21/21	2.5/2.5	2.85/2.85	Diastolic
LIMA⇒LAD	90	2.5	31/34	2.8/1.7	2/1.91	Diastolic
SVG⇒RCA	**100**	**1.5**	**5/5**	**2/1**	**10/10**	**Diastolic**
LIMA⇒LAD	85	2	11/11	1.9/1.9	7.2/7.2	Diastolic
LIMA⇒LAD	90	2.5	35/35	1.2/1.2	2.28/2.28	Diastolic
LIMA⇒D	90	2	14/31	1.8/1.3	5.8/2.5	Diastolic
RIMA⇒RCA	100	2.5	4/47	1/0.8	1.4/1.2	Diastolic
SVG⇒CX	50	1.5	22/49	3.1/2.1	2.9/1	Diastolic
SVG⇒OM	90	2.0	23/24	5/5	2.69/2.69	Diastolic
LIMA⇒LAD	90	1.5	150/150	2.3/2.3	0.53/0.53	Diastolic
SVG⇒CX	90	1.5	85/85	2.2/2.2	0.98/0.098	Diastolic
LIMA⇒LAD	**85**	**1.5**	**10/5**	**5/5**	**9/13**	**Diastolic**
SVG⇒RCA	80	2.0	15/22	2/1.8	4.33/2.9	Diastolic
LIMA⇒LAD	90	2.0	23/19	1.8/3.9	3.3/4	Diastolic
SVG⇒RCA	95	2.0	19/19	4/4	4/4	Diastolic
LIMA⇒LAD	100	1.5	28/49	5.1/3.5	2.6/1.5	Diastolic
LIMA⇒LAD	80	2.0	24/35	2.9/1	2.9/1.9	Diastolic
SVG⇒OM	80	2.5	64/64	4.1/2.9	0.9/1	Diastolic
SVG⇒OM2	90	2	18/14	3.6/5.4	3/6	Diastolic
SVG⇒RCA	100	1.0	86/63	1.8/0.7	0.8/1.18	Diastolic
SVG⇒D	90	1.5	6/6	4.6/4	11.16/11.16	Diastolic
SVG⇒OM2	100	2.5	31/32	6.2/6	1.74/1.74	Diastolic
SVG⇒LAD	90	1.5	9/19	1.8/1.9	7.4/3.5	Diastolic
LIMA⇒LAD	**50**	**1.5**	**8/6**	**3.4/2.6**	**10.3/14**	**Diastolic**
LIMA⇒LAD	90	2.0	22/31	3.5/2.7	3.5/2	Diastolic
SVG⇒LAD	60	1.5	31/31	1.6/1	1.83/1.83	Diastolic
SVG⇒CX	60	1.5	15/15	3.3/3.3	3.8/3.8	Diastolic
SVG⇒RCA	70	2.0	52/56	4/3.2	1.36/1.25	Diastolic
SVG⇒OM1	75	2.0	19/19	3/2.9	3.15/3.15	Diastolic
SVG⇒D	75	2.0	28/20	3/2.5	3/4.2	Diastolic
SVG⇒RCA	95	2.5	50/54	4.5/4	2/2	Diastolic
SVG⇒OM2	100	1.5	12/20	1.5/1	5/5	Diastolic
SVG⇒OM2	90	2.5	40/50	2/3	3/2.7	Diastolic

LIMA = left internal mammary artery; SVG = saphenous vein graft; RIMA = right mammary artery; LAD = left anterior descending; D = diagonal; RCA = right coronary artery; CX = circumflex coronary artery; OM = obtuse marginal.

is effective in detecting highly stenotic coronary anastomoses. The sensitivity of TTFM in detecting less than critical stenoses remains to be defined and is probably dependent on the surgeon's experience in correctly interpreting the flow findings. Cerrito et al.[9] have proposed a neural network pattern recognition analysis to recognize TTFM characteristics improving intraoperative detection of anastomotic errors. After a complex mathe-matical analysis of the flow curves, it is possible to detect stenoses causing a 50% or greater narrowing of the anastomoses. It is evident that less than critical stenoses cannot be detected by TTFM due to the fact that no mod-ifications in the hemodynamic performances of the grafts occur at this level. At the present time, standard or nominal curves and flow values for different types of grafts and revascularized vessels have not been de-scribed and the variability between different subjects and within subjects is extremely large.

Spence et al. have tested the ability of 19 international surgeons to de-tect anastomotic errors by evaluating mean flow and flow waveforms. More than 70% of the surgeons accepted anastomoses with severe stenoses, and all of them were able to detect highly stenotic anastomoses (>90% stenosis).[10]

The ability to correctly interpret TTFM findings needs to be slowly ac-quired, with clinical and experimental experience, and for this reason, sur-geons who have never been previously exposed to this type of technology cannot easily give the exact importance to the TTFM patterns. Correct in-terpretation of TTFM findings may be difficult if this technology is not routinely applied and established protocols and rules for flow measure-ment are not followed. Although most of the TTFM findings have an im-mediate interpretation, there is a learning curve for the most difficult cases. Confidence with the flowmeter increases with the number of cases in which this technology is applied.

In our experience, early detection of stenotic grafts can be achieved by the surgeons' simultaneous evaluation of flow patterns, PI values, flow values, and clinical findings (i.e., ECG tracing, hemodynamic values). Flow curves in patent grafts have a mainly diastolic pattern with a small component of negative systolic flow. The diastolic flow is the actual flow that at every diastole flows from the graft into the coronary artery through the anastomosis; the systolic component is retrograde flow that cannot flow into the anastomosis during systole and goes backward into the graft (Fig. 3). In the case of stenotic anastomoses, the flow curve becomes spiky and mainly systolic (Fig. 14). In this situation, the main flow through the graft is systolic and there is minimal perfusion of the anastomosis during diastole. Even if these rules apply generally to all vessels, we have noticed some differences whenever testing grafts anastomosed to the right coro-nary system. A good component of blood flow into the right coronary artery takes place during systole simply due to a minor compression of the epicardial vessels during right ventricular contraction. For this reason, a larger component of systolic positive flow can be observed in patent anas-tomoses to the RCA (Fig. 6).

Di Giammarco et al. have tried to define some nominal and objective flow and PI values for a correct interpretation of TTFM findings. Many dif-

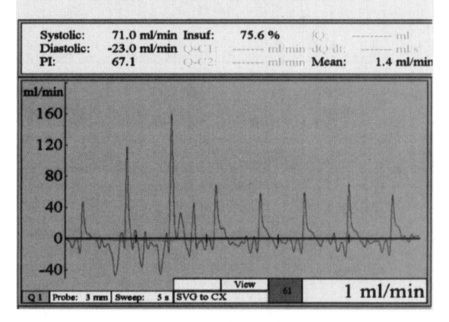

Figure 14. TTFM in a fully occluded SVG-CX.

ferences in TTFM patterns of different coronary grafts have been noted but, at the present time, no standard values have been reported.[11]

Flow value per se did not prove to be a good indicator of the quality of the anastomosis and, for this reason, graft revision cannot be justified only on the basis of absolute flow. In our experience, graft revision was erroneously performed in 3 cases only on the basis of low flow values despite satisfactory flow patterns and low PI values; at surgical inspection, no anastomotic lesions were found and the flow values remained unchanged after revision (Tables 1, 2). Use of vasodilating agents (i.e., papaverine and nitroglycerine) did not improve the flow values. In these particular cases, the small caliber of the revascularized coronary arteries (1.5 mm) and the poor quality of the distal territory were responsible for our findings (Fig. 13).

Coronary flow reserve could help in correctly diagnosing anastomotic imperfections by TTFM. In this regard, Walpoth et al. have showed how the quality of the anastomosis can be better detected by recording the modifications of flow during infusion of adenosine.[12] In this way the surgeon can easily detect the dynamic ability of the anastomoses to increase blood flow whenever oxygen requests are increased.

PI values are per se very suggestive of the quality of the anastomoses. As mentioned in the results, we correctly revised 5 grafts on the basis of abnormal flow curves and high PI values (22.04 ± 21.17 with snare and 13.94 ± 19.77 without snare) despite the fact that flow was on average higher than 15 mL/min (Fig. 8). At surgical inspection, all 5 anastomoses were shown to be severely stenotic and after revision flow patterns and PIs were improved (Fig. 9) (2.64 ± 1.07 with snare and 2.82 ± 1.01 without snare) (Tables 1, 2).

To our knowledge, an absolute PI value has never been officially proposed and we empirically decided on a limit of 5 as an absolute value on the basis of our clinical experience. Di Giammarco et al. proposed a value of 3 as the limit PI above which an anastomosis should be revised but, again, this value seems to be derived by personal clinical experience.[11]

Flow curves, PI, and mean flow values should always be evaluated with and without occlusion of the native coronary arteries (Fig. 7). The shape of the curve should remain unchanged when snaring the coronary artery proximally, and an increase in absolute flow should be recorded if competition from the native coronary artery is present with the unsnared coronary artery. The proximal snare will also permit detection of lesions at the level of the toe of the anastomosis; in this situation, whenever the coronary artery is snared, the absolute flow will drastically decrease, documenting lack of antegrade flow through the anastomosis (Fig. 12).

TTFM should be performed more times during different phases of the operation. As already mentioned, blood flow is directly proportional to systemic blood pressure and vascular resistance. In some cases, especially when arterial conduits are used, a sudden decrease in systemic pressure and excessive manipulation of the graft may cause acute spasm with consequent decrease in graft flow. This situation could lead to unnecessary revisions if appropriate TTFM measurements are not performed more times and after infusion of papaverine (Fig. 15).

Verification of intraoperative TTFM findings can be obtained with immediate postoperative angiographic studies. Angiography, per se, gives a limited bidimensional view of the coronary arteries and the coronary grafts without giving any specific information about the hemodynamic parameters of the anastomoses; for this reason, a comparative study between postoperative angiography and intraoperative TTFM may be difficult. In reoperative CABG cases, for example, we found conflicting results when comparing preoperative angiography and intraoperative TTFM; in one particular case, angiographic documentation of anastomotic subocclusion of an old saphenous graft was not confirmed during surgical revision and intraoperative TTFM.

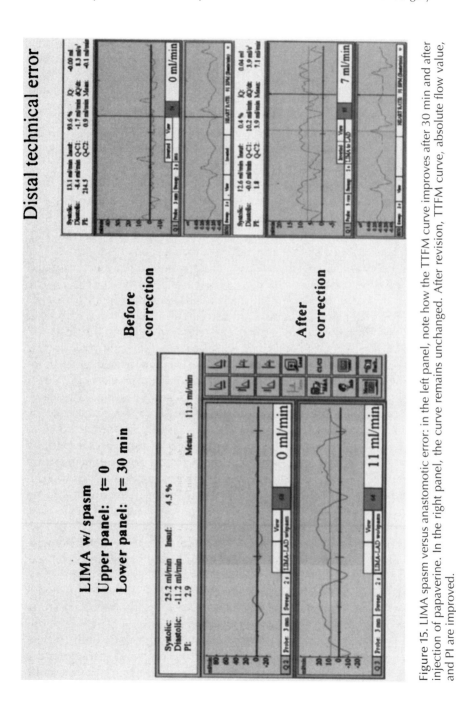

Figure 15. LIMA spasm versus anastomotic error: in the left panel, note how the TTFM curve improves after 30 min and after injection of papaverine. In the right panel, the curve remains unchanged. After revision, TTFM curve, absolute flow value, and PI are improved.

Louagie et al.[13] reported that intraoperative hemodynamic assessment via pulsed Doppler flowmeter can have a satisfactory predictive value for midterm graft occlusion. On the contrary, the same hemodynamic parameters are useless for prediction of midterm graft stenosis.

TTFM has also been compared with other techniques of postopeartive graft patency verification that, in contrast to angiography, can give more precise information about the hemodynamic characteristics of the grafts. In a series of 22 patients, Walpoth et al.[14] have shown a significant correlation between intraoperative TTFM and postoperative magnetic resonance findings of the internal mammary artery grafts.

In conclusion, there are certainly some limits in the interpretation of TTFM findings and there is still a necessity to define the sensitivity of TTFM in detecting less than critical stenoses.[8–10] Even if interpretation of graft flows is still based on personal experience and empirical values, there are no good excuses for avoiding intraoperative graft patency verification. Correct interpretation of flow curves, mean flows, and PI values are crucial in reducing the number of undetected technical errors and in decreasing the number of grafts erroneously revised. The mean flow value per se is not a good indicator of the quality of the anastomosis. Acceptable flow values with abnormal flow patterns and high PIs may identify highly stenosed anastomoses. On the contrary, low flow conditions may occur in fully patent anastomoses whenever the revascularized territory has poor runoff.

The flowmeter should be used routinely to improve patient care and surgical results independent of the surgical technique adopted; only in this way will the surgeon's ability to interpret TTFM findings improve. Graft revision should be promptly performed whenever flow curves, mean flows, and PI values are abnormal. In this situation, revision of the distal anastomoses leads to improvement in flow patterns. Postoperative outcome can be improved by meticulous use and understanding of TTFM in patients undergoing coronary artery surgery with and without CPB.

References

1. Louagie YAG, Haxhe JP, Jamarat J, Buch M, Schoevaerdts JC. Intraoperative assessment of coronary artery bypass grafts using a pulsed Doppler flowmeter. Ann Thorac Surg 1994; 58:742–749.
2. Canver CC, Dame N. Ultrasonic assessment of internal thoracic artery graft flow in the revascularized heart. Ann Thorac Surg 1994; 58:135–138.
3. Canver CC, Cooler SD, Murray EL, et al. Clinical importance of measuring coronary graft flows in the revascularized heart: ultrasonic or electromagnetic? J Cardiovasc Surg 1997; 38:211–215.
4. Walpoth BH, Bosshard A, Kipfer B, et al. Failed coronary artery bypass anastomosis detected by intraoperative coronary flow measurement. Eur J Cardiothorac Surg 1996; 10:1064–1070.

5. Jaber SF, Koenig SC, Bhasker Rao B, et al. Role of graft flow measurement technique in anastomotic quality assessment in minimally invasive CABG. Ann Thorac Surg 1998; 66:1087–1092.

6. Bergsland J, Karamanoukian HL, Soltoski PR, Salerno TA. Use of single suture technique to expose the anterior surface of the heart. J Card Surg 2000; 14(6):460–461.

7. D'Ancona G, Karamanoukian H, Ricci M , Schmid S, Spanu I, et al. Intraoperative graft verification: should you trust your fingertips? Heart Surg Forum 2000; 1898:99–102.

8. D'Ancona G, Karamanoukian H, Ricci M, Schmid S, Bergsland J, et al. Graft revision after transit time flow measurement in off-pump coronary artery bypass grafting. Eur J Cardiothorac Surg 2000; 17:287–293.

9. Cerrito PB, Koenig SC, Van Himbergen DJ, Jaber SF, et al. Neural network pattern recognition analysis of graft flow characteristics improves intraoperative anastomotic error detection in minimally invasive CABG. Eur J Cardiothorac Surg 1999; 16:88–93.

10. Jaber SF, Koenig SC, BhaskerRao B, Van Himbergen DJ, Spence PA. Can visual assessment of flow waveform morphology detect anastomotic error in off-pump coronary artery bypass grafting? Eur J Cardiothorac Surg 1998; 14:476–479.

11. Di Giammarco G. Myocardial revascularization without cardiopulmonary bypass. Presented at the symposium: State of the art in emerging coronary revascularization. EACTS, Glasgow, Scotland, Sept 4, 1999.

12. Walpoth BH, Bosshard A, Genyk I, et al. Transit time flow measurement for detection of early graft failure during myocardial revascularization. Ann Thorac Surg 1998; 66:1097–1100.

13. Louagie YAG, Brockmann CE, Jamarat J, et al. Pulsed Doppler intraoperative flow assessment and midterm coronary graft patency. Ann Thorac Surg 1998; 66:1282–1288.

14. Walpoth BH, Muller MF, Genyk I, et al. Evaluation of coronary bypass flow with color-Doppler and magnetic resonance imaging techniques: comparison with intraoperative flow measurements. Eur J Cardiothorac Surg 1999; 15:795–802.

7

Formal Flow in Coronary Surgery

Gabriele Di Giammarco, MD

Introduction

The possibility of performing intraoperative graft patency verification during coronary artery surgery has always been an unachieved objective since early experiences with myocardial revascularization. Various methods such as electromagnetic flow measurement and ultrasound velocity Doppler examination have shown important limits. A method that allows reliable and straightforward evaluation of morphofunctional parameters of coronary graft flow is undoubtedly clinically useful and represents a unique occasion to introduce some pathophysiological hypotheses.

The Coronary Flow Curve

The flow dynamics in the myocardial circulation seem to be quite different from those observed in other muscular territories. Myocardial blood flow is mainly diastolic. The flow curve shows, in normal conditions, a modulation between the "zero flow" line and the maximum flow value.

The increased myocardial oxygen demand determines a relative, but meanwhile prevalent, increase of the diastolic phase of the curve with or without change of the lowest flow value. On the other hand, in the skeletal muscle, the same situation is responsible for the variation of both the blood velocity curve and the one of the flow. This leads to a remarkable increase in the mean flow due to the upward shift of the lowest point of modulation of the curve. In this case, the curve draws a wide area of continuous flow that never reaches the "zero line. "

From: D'Ancona G, Karamanoukian HL, Ricci M, Salerno TA, Bergsland J (eds). *Intraoperative Graft Patency Verification in Cardiac and Vascular Surgery.* © Futura Publishing Company, Armonk, NY, 2001.

Transit Time Parameters of Flow

The transit time technology offers many advantages when compared to the more obsolete methods of graft patency verification. The principles of transit time flow measurement (TTFM) have been discussed in other chapters.

The parameters derived from TTFM are shown in Figure 1. From the parameters directly measured it is also possible to calculate:

- the pulsatility index (PI) according to the following formula: (Qmax-Qmin)/Qmean
- the resistance index (RI) in ohms
- the trace harmonic analysis according to fast Fourier transform.

At the beginning of our experience with TTFM, we used this technology mainly to measure the flow through all grafts performed on the beating heart. Later we extended this method to patients operated on with cardiopulmonary bypass (CPB). This was done because unavoidable technical errors (intimal flap, purse-string effect, heel or toe tapering,

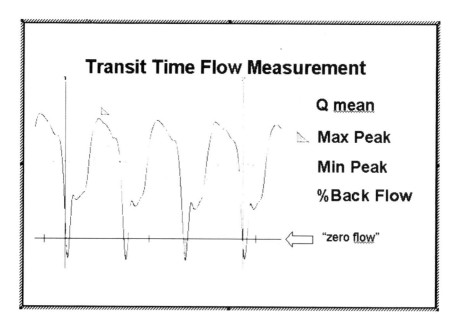

Figure 1. Transit time parameters of flow: Q mean = mean value of flow (the top horizontal line in the graph); Max Peak = maximum peak of flow above the "zero flow line"; Min peak = maximum peak of flow below the "zero flow line"; % Back Flow = % of the area of flow below the "zero flow line."

acute thrombosis) can sometimes occur in spite of conditions of perfect visibility and stability such as during cardioplegic arrest.

The availability of such technology allows a timely evaluation of the anastomosis and consequently a prompt revision in case of abnormalities. Obviously, due to its abstract and somewhat empiric value, the flow curve is to be validated.

First, we tried to understand the meaning of the parameters given by the flowmeter. We analyzed the TTFM findings in 193 patients operated on with or without CPB. We tried to define the readability of the transit time curve in the absence of perturbation of its contour, which might lead to a wrong analysis (Table 1).

We performed 354 distal anastomoses, mostly to the left anterior descending coronary artery (LAD) territory. A total of 207 internal mammary arteries (right and left) were anastomosed, preferably to the LAD territory either as in situ or as free grafts in composite conduits. The greater saphenous vein (SV) was the conduit of choice for the right coronary artery (RCA) area. We found higher absolute flow values in the LAD grafts versus the circumflex (Cx) and RCA grafts (Table 2).[1]

The TTFM technology allows measuring the amount of flow below the "zero flow" line. This component represents the backward flow through the graft. It is an area specifically called % backflow (BF) and is measured as percentage of the total area described on the trace. It could be interpreted as an indirect sign of the anastomosis patency. Furthermore, on the basis of our experience, the amount of BF seems to be inversely related to the degree of the coronary stenosis proximal to the graft.

The images reported hereafter demonstrate that the flow trace changes in response to the occlusive maneuvers performed on the coronary artery proximally or distally to the anastomotic site. The graft represented (Fig. 2) is the left internal mammary artery (LIMA) and the target

Table 1
Transit Time Flow Measurement

LAD single	164
LAD seq	29
CX single	43
CX seq	18
RCA single	91
RCA seq	9
Total samples	354 (193 pz)

The table summarizes the total number of the distal anastomoses along with their location and the fashion (single or sequential).
See text for abbreviations.

Table 2
Transit Time Flow Measurement

	Q Mean	Max Peak	Min Peak	% BFlow	PI
LAD (193)	41.48	71.72	−10.59	2.07	2.09
	(SE 1.79)°	(SE 2.99)[+]	(SE 1.01)§*	(SE 0.23)	(SE 0.05)
Cx (61)	34.93	60.85	−5.25	1.36	2.04
	(SE 2.69)	(SE 4.24)	(SE 0.95)	(SE 0.33)	(SE 0.11)
RCA (100)	33.56	60.22	−6.08	1.44	2.19
	(SE 2.06)	(SE 3.12)	(SE 0.87)	(SE 0.31)	(SE 0.13)
Total (354)	38.11	66.60	−8.40	1.77	2.11
	(SE 1.24)	(SE 2.01)	(SE 0.64)	(SE 0.16)	(SE 0.05)

Parameters of transit time flow recorded among all of the grafts analyzed according to each single coronary territory.
§ $P < .0005$.
* $P < .003$.
° $P < .006$.
+ $P < .006$.

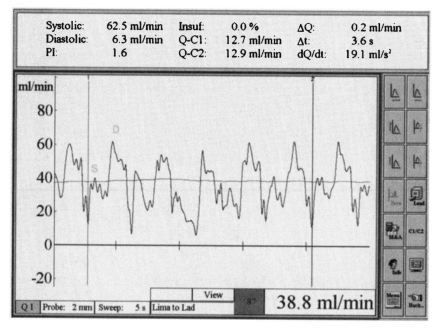

Figure 2. Transit time flow trace from a LIMA graft to the LAD after releasing the snare on the coronary artery distal to the anastomosis. S = systolic peak of flow; D = diastolic peak of flow.

vessel is the LAD coronary artery. The coronary stenosis is equal to 70%, evidently not critical in basal conditions. After the anastomosis is completed, the distal snare is released; the recorded flow trace (Fig. 2) shows a good modulation, suggesting a good anastomosis patency.

It is noteworthy to say that, immediately after the distal snare is released, the highest amount of flow is recorded. During the following few minutes, the flow values go down to what should be considered the actual flow value. This situation is a usual finding during off-pump coronary artery bypass grafting (OPCAB). This could be the evidence of the hyperemic reaction to the vessel occlusion. It can be considered as a sign of the good patency of the toe of the anastomosis. These findings mimic those obtained after infusion of a drug that increases the O_2 demand (i.e., adenosine).

After release of both snares (Fig. 3), the actual contribution of the graft to the coronary circulation is evident. All flow parameters show a reduction, and the backward flow through the graft starts to appear. In addition, the PI value reaches the upper limits of the range considered to be normal; this finding will be further analyzed later in this chapter.

Measurements after distal snare occlusion appear to be similar (Fig. 4), the only difference being a further increase in the % BF that is probably due

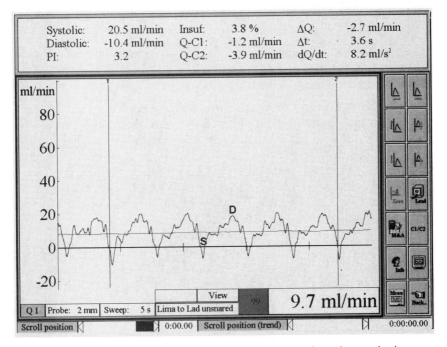

Systolic:	20.5 ml/min	Insuf:	3.8 %	ΔQ:	-2.7 ml/min	
Diastolic:	-10.4 ml/min	Q-C1:	-1.2 ml/min	Δt:	3.6 s	
PI:	3.2	Q-C2:	-3.9 ml/min	dQ/dt:	8.2 ml/s^2	

Figure 3. Transit time flow trace from a LIMA to the LAD after releasing both snares on the coronary artery across the anastomosis. S = systole onset (negative); D = diastolic peak of flow.

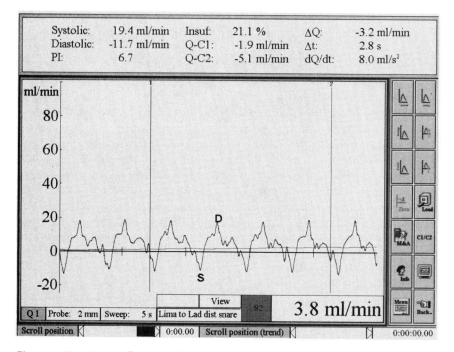

Figure 4. Transit time flow trace from a LIMA to the LAD during the coronary artery snaring distal to the anastomosis. S = systolic backward peak of flow; D = diastolic forward peak of flow.

to the actual end-to-end connection between the portion of the coronary artery proximal to the anastomosis and the graft itself. The observed increased PI value could be reasonably explained by: (1) the occlusive effect of the snare on the total balance of flow, simulating a true stenosis, and (2) the progressive increase of the backward flow through the graft during systole related to the mean flow decrease. It is clear that the control of the anastomosis patency in a similar situation could not be performed just on the basis of the basal parameters without the occlusion test described.

A PI value above 3 is commonly considered a sign of anastomotic failure. From our experience is not rare to notice even higher values along with a high % BF. On the basis of this finding, we analyzed the statistical correlation between these 2 parameters. The first step of this correlation has been performed, checking all of the anastomoses (n=354). In this case we found a positive correlation with r = 0.82 (95% confidence limits) as shown in Figure 5.[1]

As far as the 164 single anastomoses on the LAD territory are concerned, we found an even better correlation (r = 0.89) with the same confidence limits (Fig. 6).[1]

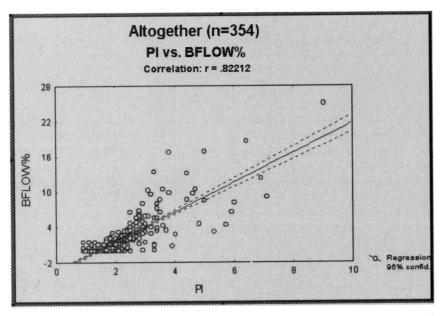

Figure 5. Correlation graph between the pulsatility index (PI) and the percentage of backward flow (%BFLOW) through all the grafts (n = 354).

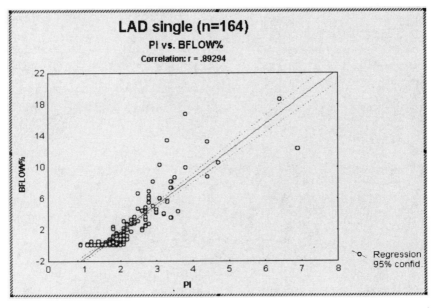

Figure 6. Correlation graph between the pulsatility index (PI) and the percentage of backward flow (%BFLOW) through all of the 164 internal mammary arteries (LIMA = 82; RIMA = 82) directed to the LAD as a single graft.

Table 3
Transit Time Flow Measurement (LAD territory—164 single anastomoses)

	LIMA	RIMA	P
Q mean	37.14 ± 24.73	46.66 ± 25.61	0.016
Max Peak	65.78 ± 40.39	79.78 ± 43.37	0.033
Min Peak	12.78 ± 16.64	9.69 ± 13.04	ns
% Backflow	2.81 ± 3.94	1.54 ± 2.49	0.015
PI	2.24 ± 1.01	2.00 ± 0.67	ns

Transit time parameters of flow recorded from 164 internal mammary artery grafts (LIMA = 82; RIMA = 82) to the LAD territory anastomosed in single fashion.
ns = not significant.
See text for abbreviations.

Furthermore, we considered the % BF on the same coronary territory analyzing the eventual difference between LIMA (n = 82) and right internal mammary artery (RIMA) (n = 82) used in 164 single distal anastomoses; the result was a higher % BF whenever the LIMA was used (Table 3).[1] This evidence could be explained by the physiological delay in the time of onset of the systolic wave in the aortic branches as we progress from the aortic valve to the iliac bifurcation.[2]

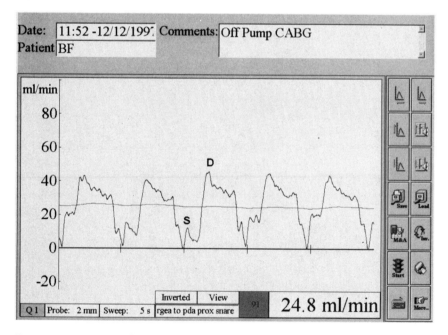

Figure 7. Transit time flow trace from the right gastroepiploic artery (RGEA) to the posterior descending artery (PDA) of the coronary artery proximal to the anastomosis. S = systolic peak of (forward) flow; D = diastolic peak of flow.

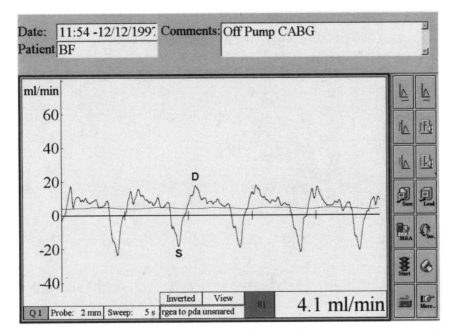

Figure 8. Transit time flow from the RGEA to the PDA after both snares are released on the coronary artery across the anastomosis. S = systolic backward peak of flow; D = diastolic forward peak of flow.

This hypothesis is somewhat confirmed by what we found recording the flow trace from the right gastroepiploic artery (RGEA) grafted on a beating heart to the posterior descending coronary artery (PDA). The trace shown in Figure 7 is recorded with the PDA proximally occluded. In this case the shape of the curve is quite similar to what we have recorded on the LAD territory, in the absence of any backward flow through the graft.

After the release of the proximal snare, the flow trace modifies with the appearance of a quite high % BF as well as a high PI (Fig. 8). If an SV graft is adopted, none of the above findings are recorded whenever the graft is proximally connected to the ascending aorta and distally anastomosed to an even less stenotic PDA.

Coming back to Table 3, there is one more interesting piece of evidence of the total amount of flow: the mean and peak flows of the RIMA anastomosed to the LAD appear significantly higher than those of the LIMA grafted on the same territory. A possible reason could be the higher prevalence, in the overall population, of right-handed people who usually show a RIMA with a larger size than the LIMA.

Another issue we tried to address is the difference, in TTFM findings, between OPCAB and traditional CABG. For our purposes, we considered just the single anastomoses (n=298) in order to make the study group ho-

Table 4
Transit Time Flow Measurement (Single anastomoses [n = 298])

		p2	Q Mean	P	Mean Peak	P	Min Peak	P	% BF	P	PI	P
LAD	CPB	82	40.11	ns	70.37	ns	12.95	ns	2.57	ns	2.20	ns
	OP	82	43.70		75.19		9.53		1.79		2.03	
Cx	CPB	22	38.94	ns	69.63	ns	6.77	ns	1.31	ns	2.30	ns
	OP	21	28.39		50.06		3.38		1.26		2.08	
RCA	CPB	47	37.28	.008	64.72	.008	5.42	ns	1.56	ns	2.03	ns
	OP	44	23.28		46.50		5.82		1.34		2.35	

Comparison between off- and on-pump transit time parameters of flow in 298 single distal anastomoses according to the 3 main territories.
CPB = cardiopulmonary bypass CABG; OP = off-pump CABG; ns = not significant.

mogeneous for all of the 3 territories analyzed. The results are summarized in Table 4.[1]

The only difference was found on the RCA territory where the flow values recorded during on-pump CABG were significantly higher than after OPCAB. In our opinion, this might be due either to the release of vasoactive substances after CPB or to the infusion of vasoconstrictive drugs normally adopted to control blood pressure during OPCAB.

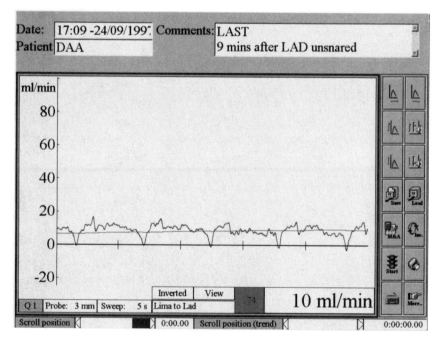

Figure 9. Transit time flow trace from a LIMA grafted to an LAD supplying a high resistance territory. The measurement was taken 9 minutes after both snares were released.

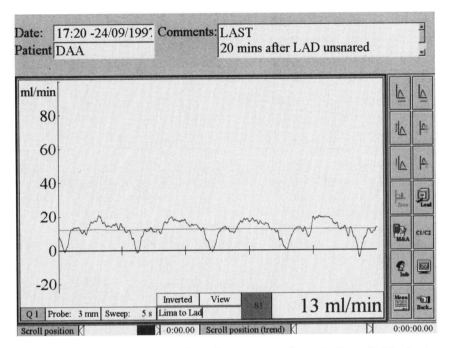

Figure 10. Transit time flow trace from the same case shown in Figure 9, 20 minutes after the LAD snares were released.

A common question arising when a flow measurement method is discussed concerns the amount of flow considered to be acceptable in order to ensure a good function of the graft. The quantitative flow evaluation of the transit time method is demonstrated to be very close to the real value.[3] In our opinion, a low flow through the anastomosis is to be considered a sign of failure only if it is not possible to record a well-modulated flow trace. In other words, the shape of the trace seems to be highly important in evaluating the anastomosis patency, especially whenever TTFM is performed in patent grafts anastomosed to coronary artery branches with a high vascular resistance (previous transmural myocardial necrosis). Reported in Figure 9 is a case of a LIMA-to-LAD single anastomosis performed on a beating heart via minimal access. The amount of flow recorded just after having performed the anastomosis reveals a low value together with a well-modulated trace. The repeated measurement taken 20 minutes later shows a 30% increase of the flow value (Fig. 10).

Morphology of the Trace

The flow trace is undoubtedly the most intriguing and open issue of the transit time flow measurement. The diastolic phase of the curve modifies together with the quality of the coronary artery target. Three different situations may present in the revascularized vessel:

1. subcritical stenosis
2. critical stenosis
3. vessel occlusion in presence of:
   a. no infarcts
   b. previous myocardial necrosis.

The information derived is easier to interpret when the graft–coronary artery is considered as a unit. The diastolic trace of the flow curve should also be considered together with the systolic component, which may represent the keypoint for detecting subcritical stenoses. The accepted flow trace morphology of a believed well-functioning graft shows a diastolic peak of flow higher than the systolic one.

If a segmental sampling is taken at different levels of an in situ mammary artery graft to the LAD, the prevalence of the diastolic flow peak reduces progressively when the measurement is performed closer to the origin of the internal mammary artery. On the contrary, the global mean flow is unchanged. This could be due to the distance between the measurement site and the subclavian artery.

Analog findings are obtained whenever transthoracic pulsed wave (PW) Doppler is used to detect graft patency after LIMA-to-LAD revascularization via a left anterior small thoracotomy (LAST).[4,5] At the level of the second or third intercostal space, the morphology of the PW Doppler trace (Fig. 11 a,b) recorded postoperatively is very similar to the transit time flow trace recorded intraoperatively at the level of the LIMA-LAD anastomosis (Fig. 12).

When the IMA is checked above the clavicle, the PW Doppler shows a prevalent systolic modulation (Fig. 13). Similar findings are observed with intraoperative TTFM. This morphological analogy, beyond the different meaning of the 2 traces, could be useful to follow-up the in situ internal mammary arteries after the operation.

Validation of the Method

Flowmetry in coronary surgery has recently gained popularity following the renewed interest in OPCAB. Technical improvements have allowed new methods of flowmetry to become available in the daily surgical armamentarium. In addition, the transit time flowmeters have been used to validate the quality of the beating heart anastomoses. With the use of such an instrument, however, the attention of the surgeon has

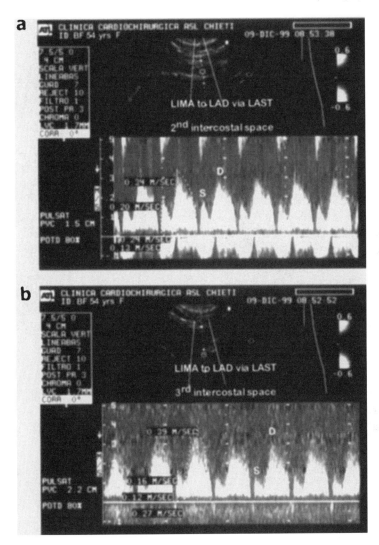

Figure 11. Pulsed wave (PW) echo–2D Doppler velocity of flow evaluation from a LIMA grafted to the LAD via a left anterior small thoracotomy (LAST operation). (a) LIMA detected at the level of second intercostal space. (b) LIMA detected at the level of the third intercostal space.

been more focused on the quality control of the anastomosis per se, whatever technique is used to construct it. This concept is particularly true after the improvements achieved in the OPCAB that have led to better results, comparable to those obtained with the standard technique.[6] That is why in our clinical practice we decided to routinely extend the

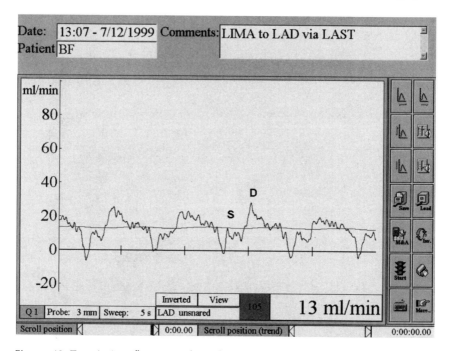

Figure 12. Transit time flow trace from the same patient as in Figure 11. The morphological analogy with the PW Doppler finding is evident. S = systolic peak of flow; D = diastolic peak of flow.

flow measurement to all coronary grafts performed independently from the surgical strategy.

According to this opinion, the TTFM meets the need for intraoperative quality control of the anastomosis, especially whenever an angiogram cannot be performed.[7] Quality control should be performed to guarantee prompt graft revision if the criteria of patency are not met.[8–10]

On the basis of these statements, it is necessary to compare the method with angiography, the presumed "gold standard" for anastomotic quality assessment. We analyzed, for this purpose, the flow traces derived from the LIMA grafts to the LAD in 25 patients revascularized without CPB and submitted early postoperatively to control angiography. The analysis was performed by evaluating a single heartbeat for each patient and averaging every single instantaneous sample having the same time relationship with all 25 beats, with the aim of observing the morphology of the reconstructed flow trace. The criteria as the basis of the analysis are reported as follows:

- All measurements were performed after proximal and distal snaring technique.

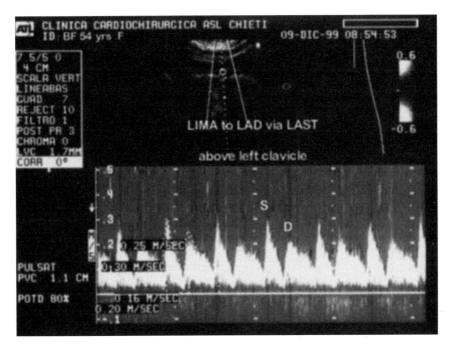

Figure 13. PW echo–2D Doppler velocity of flow detection of the same in situ LIMA as in Figures 11 and 12. The probe is placed above the left clavicle in order to record the trace close to the origin of the graft from the subclavian artery. S = systolic velocity peak; D = diastolic velocity peak.

- The probes were placed on the LIMA close to the anastomosis.
- Probes with the same sampling frequency (i.e., samples have the same time spacing) were used.
- One representative heartbeat was analyzed within a stable measurement of more than 10 seconds.
- Measurements were taken just after completion of the anastomosis.
- Time axis was standardized to include all patients with a heart rate within ± 10% of the mean value (=75 beats/min).

The modulation of the generated trace overlapped that of the trace we believed to be normal. The matched control angiographies revealed in all cases the perfect patency of all the 25 anastomoses (Fig. 14).[1] Even if the analysis refers to the LIMA-to-LAD anastomosis, it is reasonable to hypothesize that following the same criteria, it is possible to obtain similar traces from the circumflex (Cx) territories.

On the other hand, there is some uncertainty concerning the flow traces recorded from the RCA territory. In this case we recorded either a flow trace similar to that previously reported or a mainly systolic one, al-

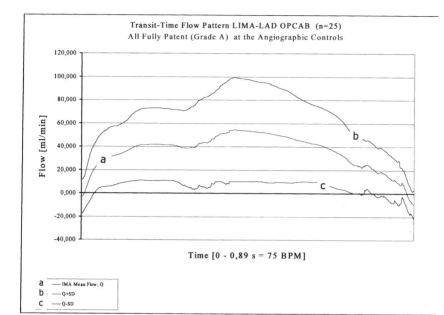

Figure 14. Transit time flow-generated trace according to the criteria defined in the text.

ways in the presence of full angiographic patency. The possible reasons are hypothesized as follows:

- *RCA anatomy*: it is a monopodial artery giving rise to 90° angle branches, different from the left coronary circulation, with a sometimes noticeable caliber mismatch between the mainstem and the collaterals; this could lead to a heavier request of compliance to the graft implanted.
- *RCA wall condition*: it is usually the most diseased coronary artery to be grafted; the calcified wall may contribute to the previous situation.
- *Graft caliber mismatch*: the most used graft in the RCA territory is the SVG that is, quite often, much bigger than the PDA.

All of these conditions produce a flow trace with a prevalent systolic peak even if the total area, and therefore the mean flow, is within the normal values.

As mentioned above, the degree of the stenosis of the target coronary artery highly influences either the trace morphology or the parameters of flow.

In the case of a LIMA grafted to a coronary artery with mild stenosis, the flow trace will show minimal contribution of the graft to the coronary

circulation in the basal condition with a slight increase during pharmacological stimulation. The systolic flow peak will be reversed, and the diastolic flow and the total mean flow will be quite minimal.

As described above, the PI in this situation will rise well beyond the
value of 3, simulating a high resistance downward from the graft. It would
be of interest to assess to what extent this index could be meaningful in
terms of graft patency prognosis.

The flow trace recorded on a graft located distally to a severe stenosis
is the one supposed to be the standard. Some difference is evident in the
case of a complete occlusion of the target coronary vessel in the presence
of a high resistance distal territory. This is a common finding when the
LIMA revascularizes an LAD in a patient with a previous wide anterior
myocardial necrosis.

In Figure 15 the flow trace recorded from a LIMA-to-LAD graft in a
patient submitted to the excision of an apical left ventricular aneurysm is
shown. Just immediately after the CPB weaning, a low mean flow was
recorded; the repeated measurement 45 minutes later revealed a doubling
of the value.

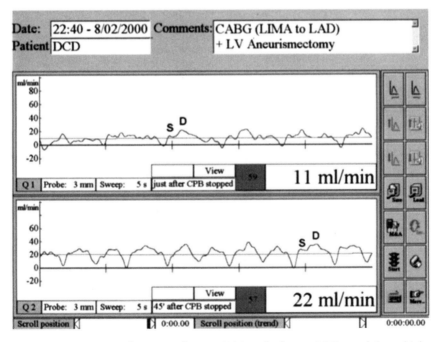

Figure 15. Transit time flow trace from a LIMA grafted to an LAD supplying a high-
resistance territory due to an extensive myocardial necrosis exiting in an LV apical
aneurysm. The upper trace was recorded just after the CPB weaning; the lower, 45
minutes after. S = systolic peak of flow; D = diastolic peak of flow.

Functional Tests

If there are almost no doubts in recognizing the transit time flow trace of an occluded graft or a severely impaired anastomosis, it is very difficult to decode subcritical stenoses[11] by means of basal measurement only. In addition, at the present time, there is lack of information about the characteristics of the systolic phase of the transit time trace. Once clarified, this information might improve the detection of less than critical stenoses.

Moreover, the heel or toe occlusion at the site of the anastomosis does not usually affect the measurement and can lead to a false negative result.

Therefore, in our clinical practice we use some functional tests: *occlusive maneuvers* and *pharmacological testing*.

In order to perform the occlusion test, 2 snaring sutures are needed across the anastomotic site[.1] This is more commonly used during off-pump coronary surgery, because this is a frequently used method to control the bleeding while suturing. The snares are gently tied to avoid any coronary damage, which is actually never observed in our practice. Once

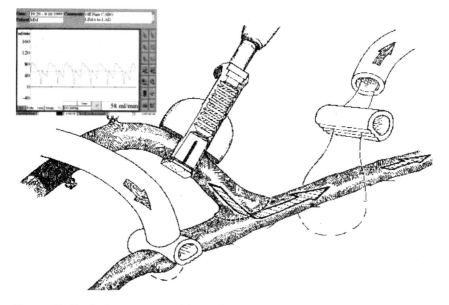

Figure 16. Occlusive maneuver. The graft–coronary artery unit is represented with the snare tightened proximal to the anastomosis. The transit time probe is represented around the graft. In the upper left corner the transit time trace of the downward flow is shown.

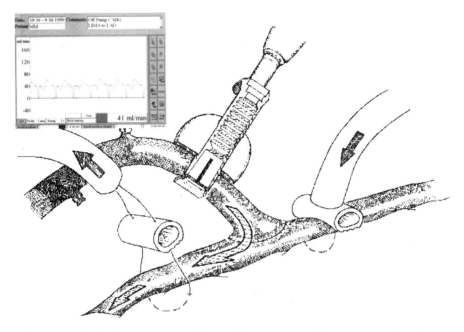

Figure 17. Occlusive maneuver. The proximal snare on the coronary artery is released while the distal snare is tightened. The transit time flow trace registered from the graft is shown in the upper left corner.

the anastomosis is complete, the distal snare is released and the flow trace is recorded to verify the toe patency (Fig. 16). As a second step, the proximal snare is released while the distal snare is tightened again. Through the flow trace recording the patency of the heel is explored (Fig. 17). Both snares are then released, showing the bidirectional anastomosis performance (Fig. 18).

The other functional test is performed using drugs that increase the flow through the anastomosis by means of increased myocardial O_2 consumption. In such a situation, the sensitivity of the transit time flow measurement improves, giving a better chance to detect restrictive anastomoses.

Among the usable drugs, we choose dobutamine because it is easy and comfortable to use. Our protocol is the continuous infusion of the drug at a dose of 5 μg/kg/min for 3 minutes or 20 μg/kg as a bolus injection. Beyond the systemic arterial pressure increase, not seen in all cases, an increase of the flow values, sometimes over 100% from the baseline, is usually recorded (Fig. 19).

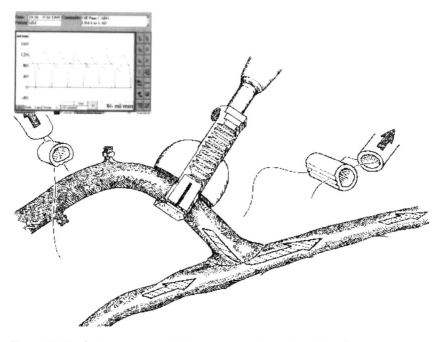

Figure 18. Occlusive maneuver. Both snares are released and the relative transit time flow trace is shown in the upper left corner.

Conclusions

It is difficult to draw any conclusions because the method is new and leaves many unanswered questions on the matter of the available parameters. In addition, the readability of the data is a direct function of the precision of their collection, sometimes not as easy as it should be. The coupling probe vessel is a decisive variable, and in our experience was reached by the use of an underestimated probe caliber.

Finally, the software commonly available is not as user-friendly as one would expect from an instrument that has to be quickly managed in the operating theater; this sometimes influences either the collection of data or their post-processing.

Regarding the advantages, it has to be said that the transit time flow measurement contributes to fill the existing gap between the preoperative evaluation and the postoperative angiography.

It should be mentioned, on the other hand, that the quality of the given information is not only morphological but also functional; this usually generates some skepticism, as its meaning is not comparable to any standard preoperative examination.

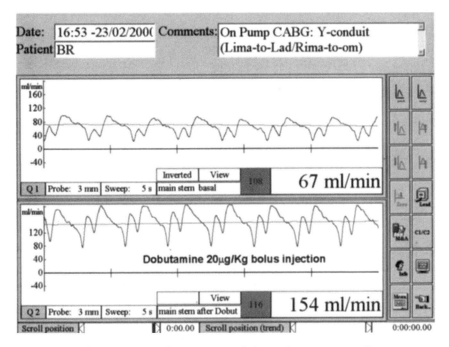

Figure 19. Dobutamine test. The upper panel shows the transit time flow measurement from the main stem of a Y-conduit (in situ LIMA-free RIMA) before the drug infusion; in the lower part, the transit time flow measurement is recorded after dobutamine infusion at a dose of 20 μg/kg as a single bolus.

The readability of the transit time flow parameters should increase in order to draw, whenever possible, from beyond the single surgeon's experience, information about the perioperative intracoronary hemodynamics using a fast, reproducible, and relatively noninvasive technology. This achievement should direct the focus of the coronary surgeon from the concept of anatomical revascularization to that of functional revascularization.

Thus far, there are still some doubts in interpreting with certainty the results of measurements. Consequently, this uncertainty on one hand leads the surgeon to have faith in the method, and on the other hand represents undoubtedly a challenge for interesting pathophysiological speculations.

References

1. Di Giammarco G. Myocardial revascularisation without cardiopulmonary bypass. Presented at the 13th Annual Meeting of the EACTS. Glasgow, Scotland. September 1999.

2. Milnor WR. Cardiovascular Physiology. Oxford University Press, 1990.
3. Matre K, Birkeland S, Hessevik I, Segadal L. Comparison of transit-time and Doppler ultrasound methods for measurement of flow in aortocoronary bypass grafts during cardiac surgery. Thorac Cardiovasc Surg 1994; 42(3): 170–174.
4. Calafiore AM, Di Giammarco G, Teodori G, Bosco G, D'Annunzio E, et al. Left anterior descending coronary artery grafting via left anterior small thoracotomy without cardiopulmonary bypass. Ann Thorac Surg 1996; 61:1658–1665.
5. Calafiore AM, Gallina S, Iacò A, Teodori G, Iovino T, et al. Minimally invasive mammary artery Doppler flow velocity evaluation in minimally invasive coronary operations. Ann Thorac Surg 1998; 66–68:1236–1241.
6. Contini M, Iacò AL, Iovino T, Teodori G, Di Giammarco G, et al. Current results in off-pump surgery. Eur J Cardiothorac Surg 1999; 16(suppl 1):S69–S72.
7. Repossini A, Moriggia S, Cianci V, Parodi O, Sganzerla P, et al. The LAST operation is safe and effective: MIDCABG clinical and angiographic evaluation. Ann Thorac Surg 2000; 70:74–78.
8. Walpoth BH, Bosshard A, Genyk I, Kipfer B, Berdat PA, et al. Transit time flow measurement for detection of early graft failure during myocardial revascularization. Ann Thorac Surg 1998; 66:1097–1100.
9. Ricci M, Karamanoukian HL, Salerno TA, D'Ancona G, Bergsland J. Role of coronary graft flow measurement during reoperations for early graft failure after off-pump coronary revascularization. J Cardiac Surg 1999; 14(5):342–347.
10. D'Ancona G, Karamanoukian HL, Ricci M, Schmid S, Bergsland J, et al. Graft revision after transit time flow measurement in off-pump coronary artery bypass grafting. Eur J Cardiothorac Surg 2000; 17(3):287–293.
11. Jaber SF, Koenig SC, Bhasker Rao B, Van Himbergen DJ, Cerrito PB, et al. Role of graft flow measurement technique in anastomotic quality assessment in minimally invasive CABG. Ann Thorac Surg 1998; 66:1087–1092.

8

Automated Classification Procedures and Neural Network Models to Predict the Level of Anastomotic Stenosis in Off-Pump CABG Surgery

Patricia B. Cerrito, PhD, Steven C. Koenig, PhD,
Paul A. Spence, MD

Introduction

Anastomotic quality has become a critical issue in off-pump coronary artery bypass graft (OPCABG) surgery, especially during minimally invasive (mini-CABG) procedures. It is very important to detect the construction of a "poor" anastomosis during the primary surgery so that repeat operations may be avoided. Several methods of intraoperative anastomotic quality assessment have been developed to help verify graft patency. One of the most common methods for assessing anastomotic quality during CABG is the measurement of graft flow(s) using clinically approved transit time flow probes (Transonics Systems, Ithaca, NY). Theory and perioperative measurements have suggested that adequate blood flow and velocity through the graft are required for long-term patency.[1-3] Transit time flow probes provide a mean flow and continuous flow waveform with good resolution (100 Hz) and accuracy.[4-6] However, the efficacy of this method has not been well established.

Some investigators have been unable to correlate graft flow with clinical outcome.[7,8] They have relied on mean flow values perioperatively to determine whether the graft will provide adequate long-term patency. In addition, surgeons may use visual assessment of flow waveforms to help

From: D'Ancona G, Karamanoukian HL, Ricci M, Salerno TA, Bergsland J (eds). *Intraoperative Graft Patency Verification in Cardiac and Vascular Surgery.* © Futura Publishing Company, Armonk, NY, 2001.

determine whether the graft is patent. However, this method has been shown to be unreliable and may lead to the acceptance of faulty anastomoses by surgeons.[9] Due to the peculiar physiology of the coronary circulation, flow through the coronary grafts occurs primarily during diastole with a short systolic peak. Absence of diastolic flow may be indicative of an occluded graft, which should serve as a warning to the surgeon to consider revising the graft. In a graft that is not occluded, but still has some degree of stenosis, the flow may be predominantly diastolic, but may exhibit taller systolic peaks. The decision of whether to revise these anastomoses intraoperatively can be difficult, particularly anastomoses containing intermediate degrees of stenosis (50–90%).

In a survey conducted by our group,[9] international experts in the field of cardiothoracic surgery were unable to use visual assessment of flow morphology or mean flows, or both, to detect certain levels of anastomotic error (Fig. 1). Virtually all surgeons were able to detect nearly occluded coronary grafts and most could identify those that were fully patent. However, there was a high failure rate in the ability to detect severe degrees of anastomotic stenosis. The ability to detect severely stenotic grafts would be extremely valuable to the surgeon because these grafts are likely to require anastomotic revision. In some instances where there is a high mean flow and/or high diastolic-to-systolic flow ratio, typically indicative of a patent graft, the anastomosis may be less than ideal. Similarly, in some cases where there is a low mean graft flow and/or low diastolic-to-systolic flow ratio, typically indicative of a poor graft, the graft may be perfectly patent. Subsequently, interpretation of anastomotic quality as a function of mean graft flow and flow waveform morphology may be difficult to establish. This may help explain why investigators have been unable to correlate mean graft flow with clinical outcome.

Mean graft flow and/or flow waveform morphology appears to be an acceptable technique for identifying patent and occluded grafts. However, these measurements do not allow the surgeon to reliably distinguish among intermediate levels of stenosis (50–90%) in grafts. We concluded that evaluation of anastomotic quality based on mean flow and flow waveform morphology alone was insufficient, and that in order to identify intermediate stenotic grafts, additional information was required. In this chapter, we present a mathematical technique, automated classification using a neural network model, that processes mean flow, flow waveform morphology characteristics, and spectral analysis of graft flow using transit time probe technology to more reliably distinguish intermediate stenotic grafts. The method was applied to 27 mongrel dogs (25–35 kg) to determine whether the level of stenosis could be predicted through the use of neural network analysis.

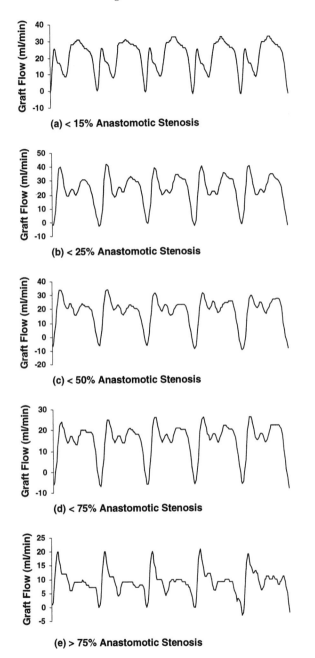

Figure 1. Flow morphology at different levels of anastomotic stenosis.

Automated Classification

It has been demonstrated that the use of an automated classification can improve the accuracy of diagnosis, particularly reducing the false negative rate.[10–12] Unless a flow tracing can be identified with an exact pattern, it becomes difficult to classify. Because of the substantial variability between individuals, it is rare to get an exact pattern in the tracing. An automated process is capable of detecting these "fuzzy" patterns and classifying them.

As stated in Swenson[13]:

As with virtually all clinical syndromes, there are 2 basic approaches to the diagnostic evaluation, with the majority of diagnostic decision-making being based on history and clinical presentation. The first approach could be termed *the red flag approach*, in which certain historical and clinical clues are elicited to assess the probability of serious disease.

The second approach to diagnosis could be termed *the pattern recognition approach*. This requires the clinician to match the patient's history and findings with a clinical picture of the various diagnostic possibilities. Based on the probabilities determined from such an analysis, additional testing may be suggested to document the existence of the condition. It also may lead to a trial of therapy for the specific disorder that, if successful, further validates the diagnosis.

Pattern recognition and classification can be valuable diagnostic tools, but there is a considerably high false negative (and/or false positive) rate that can cause problems, particularly when either type of false conclusion has serious impact on the patient. A standard type of automated classification technique is logistic regression, in which several input variables are used to predict outcomes. Unfortunately, there is low sensitivity or specificity when logistic regression is applied to images and to unfiltered time series.

One of the major drawbacks with an automatic process for reading the results of the flow measurement is that the initial starting time is not necessarily known. The time zero point can occur at the peak systolic or diastolic value, or at any point in between. This can add a substantial amount of "noise" into the time series. Therefore, initially, the results of the flow measurements are filtered through a spectral analysis.[14] Using the phase and magnitude of each harmonic value of the spectral analysis, the peaks and valleys corresponding to the systolic and diastolic points in the time series can be aligned and examined regardless of the starting time point. This prefiltering eliminates the unnecessary noise that can confuse the results of a neural network analysis.

Spectral Analysis

Any repeating time domain waveform, in this case coronary graft flow, can be represented by a Fourier series, which is a sum of cosines and sines of differing magnitudes and phase angles at integer frequencies (harmonics).[15,16] The magnitude and phase information at all frequencies, commonly referred to as the spectral content, is determined by performing a Fourier transform of the flow waveform. Using this frequency domain information (magnitudes and phases), it is often possible to identify important waveform characteristics that cannot easily be seen in the time domain waveform, thereby providing additional information to better distinguish degrees of stenosis in coronary grafts.

Mathematically, the Fourier transform of a function f(x) is equal to

$$F(s) \int_{-\infty}^{\infty} f(x) \exp\left(-i2\pi xs\right)dx$$

so that

$$f(x) = \int_{-\infty}^{\infty} \left[\int_{-\infty}^{\infty} F(s) \exp(i2\pi xs)dx \right] \exp(i2pxs)ds$$

The functions of waveforms can be split into even and odd components so that

$$f(x) = Even(x) + Odd\,(x)$$
$$Even(x) = \tfrac{1}{2}[f(x) + f\,(2x)]$$
$$Odd(x) = \tfrac{1}{2}[f(x) - f(-x)]$$

The Fourier transform then reduces to

$$2\int_{0}^{\infty} Even(x)\cos(2\pi xs)dx - 2i\int_{0}^{\infty} \sin(2\pi xs)dx$$

The general form of a spectral analysis function (using the infinite sum to approximate the integrals) is equal to

$$x_t = a_0 + \Sigma \, \{a_k \cos(\lambda_k^* \, t) + b_k \sin(\lambda_k^* \, t)\}$$

where the series of constants $\{a_k\}$ and $\{b_k\}$ must be estimated. The summation is carried out as far as it is meaningful: typically 5 terms (that is, $k=5$) because most of the spectral information resides in these terms. Since it is a relatively complex and time-consuming task to estimate these constants, an improved algorithm called the fast Fourier transform was developed.[17] It greatly improves the speed of the computations while requiring that the number of observations in the series must equal a power of 2. Since the flow probe results are relatively continuous, this requirement is not detrimental to the computations.

We were able to compare the magnitude and phase components of graft flow waveforms at different harmonics and determine significant similarities or differences.[14] Spectral analysis of the flow tracings resulted in the detection of significant differences between patent and moderately severe stenotic anastomoses, patent and severely stenotic anastomoses, and mild and moderately stenotic anastomoses.[14] Collectively, these findings provided additional information for characterizing varying degrees of anastomotic stenosis that could not be detected using traditional time domain techniques (Fig. 2). However, the spectral analysis technique could not definitively and reliably distinguish intermediate anastomotic stenoses. Subsequently, another automated classification technique, neural network analysis, was developed.

Neural Network Analysis

A neural network is a connected network of processing elements called neurons.[18] A neuron receives input values, represented typically as real numbers, on multiple input lines and computes a weighted sum on them. The neuron then uses the sum to compute an activation or threshold value. The activation value is passed to an output line, which may in turn be passed as input to another neuron or may represent the final output of the network. A typical computational neuron is depicted in Figure 3.

A group of neurons, arranged in interconnected layers and with judiciously chosen interconnection weights, can perform useful computations. Some neurons accept input from the environment, others perform internal (hidden) calculations, and still others present the final result of the network's cogitation. Some neurons may be used not to process input data, but to provide bias activation for other neurons (Fig. 4).

Given a set of input data (that is, flow measurements) $X_1, X_2, \ldots, X_n$, a competitive layer $Y_1, Y_2, \ldots, Y_m$ is defined. For each neuron Y_i in the competitive layer, a set of incoming connection weights $W_i = (W_{i1}, W_{i2}, \ldots, W_{in})$

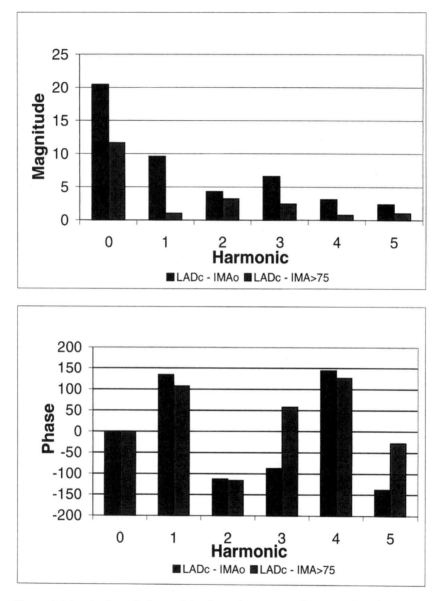

Figure 2. Magnitude and phase of the first 6 harmonics of a spectral analysis using the fast Fourier transform.

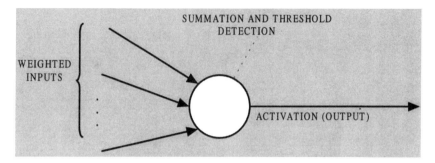

Figure 3. Diagram of a neuron in a neural network analysis.

is defined. The distance from the input X_i is defined by:

$$Distance_i = \sqrt{\sum_{j=1}^{n} (X_j - W_{ij})^2}$$

The value Y_c with the minimal distance is the chosen competitive neuron. This value is used to modify the weights such that:

$$\Delta W_{ij} = a(X_j - W_{ij}) \frac{\sin D_{ci}}{2D_{ci}}$$

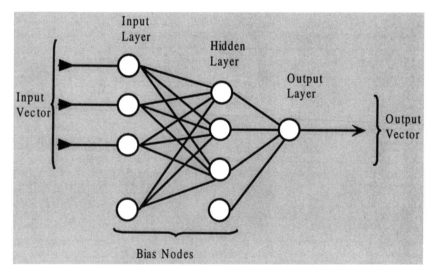

Figure 4. Diagram of a neural network analysis.

where D_{ci} is defined as the distance from the current neuron Y_i to the competitive neuron Y_c and α is a learning rate value, typically ranging from 0.2 to 0.5. Only values of Y_i located in the neighborhood of Y_c are changed. The value of α decreases by:

$$a_t = a_0 \left(1 - \frac{t}{T} \right)$$

where a_0 is the starting value at time zero, t denotes the current learning rate value, and T is the total number of passes through the data.

Judiciously choosing neural network interconnection weights is a complex task, usually accomplished by training the network. A series of example cases and target outputs are presented to the network, with the expectation that the network will begin to associate properties of the inputs with specific outputs.

When the training phase has been completed, the network is then tested in a validation or acceptance phase. There, it attempts to successfully classify data not previously used in training. At this time, the classifications produced by the network may be compared to the classifications produced by other statistical methods. Ultimately, if the network demonstrates that it can generalize over the training and validation data adequately, it may be selected for use in a production phase. Production data are entirely novel to the network and mark the encounter between the network and the real world.

Just as certain living nerve cells appear to be highly selective in responding to stimuli, so too a successfully trained neural network can be quite selective in identifying patterns. In a fully connected network, each neuron in the hidden layer receives a signal from all the input neurons, each input signal weighted by its importance. When all (or most) of the highly weighted input signals are active, the hidden-layer neuron's threshold will be crossed, causing the neuron to emit a large activation signal. Each hidden-layer neuron will, in general, have different weight patterns affecting its input lines, meaning that different overall patterns of data presented to the input neurons will be flagged by the strong activation of a corresponding hidden-layer neuron. Each hidden-layer neuron, in effect, becomes sensitive to a specific pattern of features in the input and signals the presence of the pattern by a strong activation.

Clinical Application

Forty-six patent (<15% stenosis) left and/or right internal mammary artery (IMA) grafts to LAD were constructed. Transit time flow probes

Table 1
Comparison of Analysis Methods on Training Set

Measurement	Neural Network Analysis	Logistic Regression
Sensitivity	98.6%	86%
Specificity	82.1%	35%
Positive Predictive Value	93.5%	80%
Negative Predictive Value	95.8%	45%
Accuracy	94.1%	73%

(Model 3SB, Transonic Systems Inc., Ithaca, NY) placed on the graft(s) were used to measure graft flow. Continuous beat-to-beat graft flow was recorded with the LAD occluded and the graft to LAD anastomosis under patent (<15%), mild (<25%), moderate (<50%), moderately severe (<75%), and severe (>75%) stenosis conditions. One-minute datasets containing graft flow (Q), arterial pressure (AoP), and ECG were analog-to-digital (A/D) converted, sampled at 100 Hz, and recorded using a MacLAB data acquisition system (MacLAB, Milford, MA) during each experimental condition. The degree of anastomotic stenosis was determined by random postoperative angiography.

With the use of the graft flow physiological parameters (mean flow and graft flow morphology) and the application of spectral analysis to the graph flow data, a neural network was built and tested to help improve anastomotic error detection. Our neural network was trained to estimate high or low patency at a cutpoint value of 50%. This value was used to represent an "acceptable" anastomosis of less than 50% stenosis, or an anastomosis that "should be redone" with a stenosis greater than 50%.

A random sample of 80% of the data was used as the training set in the neural network with the remaining 20% used to validate the results. The outcome from the neural network was compared to the outcome from the standard logistic regression (Table 1) in the training set and then compared in the testing set (Table 2). The neural network is far superior in

Table 2
Comparison of Analysis Methods on Validation Set

Measurement	Neural Network Analysis	Logistic Regression
Sensitivity	73%	88%
Specificity	84%	30%
Positive Predictive Value	73%	80%
Negative Predictive Value	84%	43%
Accuracy	80%	76%

specificity and in its negative predictive value. Therefore, the use of the neural network can improve on the prediction of grafts with more or less than 50% patency.[19] The automated procedure is particularly useful in reducing the proportion of false negatives so that the surgeon can focus on the patients with 50% or more stenosis.

Perspective

The neural network was shown to be very accurate in the estimation of anastomotic quality. However, this study involved hemodynamic data from canine models and needs to be applied to a human study for any future clinical applications. Although the results of the study in dogs are encouraging, it must be realized that there may be other important variables that are excluded such as initial coronary artery disease.

An issue that may cause limitations or problems in anastomotic quality assessment using transit time flowmetry is competitive flow. Competitive flow to a grafted coronary artery causes retrograde graft flow that may have a significant effect on both mean graft flow and flow waveform morphology.[20-24] In the previously mentioned studies reported by our group, the graft flows were recorded with the proximal LAD snared to avoid the effects of competitive flow on graft flow physiology. However, if used intraoperatively without snaring of the proximal coronary artery, competitive flow may alter the ability of the surgeon to assess the quality of the anastomosis. In fact, unreported studies by our group have shown that competitive flow may give misleading information to the surgeon regarding graft patency. In instances when graft flow was measured in a fully patent graft undergoing competitive flow, a taller systolic peak could appear when diastolic flow seemed diminished. In addition, when graft flow was measured in a severely stenotic graft undergoing competitive flow, diastolic flow appeared more prominent, giving the surgeon a false perception of a "good" quality anastomosis. Therefore, surgeons may wish to use extra caution when assessing graft patency when the native vessel is not occluded.

An additional important variable that needs to be addressed is the effect of distal coronary artery disease on graft flow. Unfortunately, studies are limited involving the effects of distal disease on coronary graft flow. All of these grafts were pedicled internal thoracic artery (ITA) grafts. The flow pattern of a free graft from the aorta may be considerably different. Subsequently, it is likely that an entirely different model would have to be developed to clinically evaluate these grafts.

However, these variables can be examined by using the neural network analysis to estimate the overall accuracy, sensitivity, and specificity of the transit time flow probe to predict level of stenosis. Despite the limitations of the methodology, the future clinical implications of automated classification procedures and neural network models lies in the development of a clinical database of graft flow measurements correlated to varying degrees of anastomotic stenosis, validated by angiography. In turn, these data would be used in the development of a device that assesses a graft flow waveform in real-time and quickly alerts the surgeon to the graft's patency or lack thereof.

Acknowledgment: Funding support for this project has been provided by the Jewish Hospital Heart and Lung Institute. The authors wish to thank Stan Goldman, PhD, for his editorial review of this manuscript. The authors also wish to thank Calvin Miracle for providing the artwork in Figures 3 and 4.

References

1. Walker JA, Friedberg HD, Flemma RH, Johnson WD. Determinants of angiographic patency of aortocoronary vein bypass grafts. Circ J Am Heart Assoc 1972; 45(suppl I):I-86.
2. Folts JD, Kahn DR, Bittar N, Rowe GG. Effects of partial obstruction on phasic flow in aortocoronary grafts. Circ J Am Heart Assoc 1975; 52(suppl I):I-148.
3. Gema AS, Krone RJ, McCormick JR, Baue AE. Selection of coronary bypass: anatomic physiological and angiographic considerations of vein and mammary artery grafts. J Thorac Cardiovasc 1975; 70:416.
4. Lundell A., Bergqvist D, Mattsson E, et al. Volume blood flow measurements with a transit time flowmeter: an in vivo and in vitro variability and validation study. Clin Physiol 1993; 13:547–557.
5. Canver CC, Dame NA. Ultrasonic assessment of internal thoracic artery graft in the revascularized heart. Ann Thorac Surg 1994; 58:135–138.
6. Laustsen J, Pedersen EM, Terp K, Steinbruchel D, Kure HH, et al. Validation of a new transit time ultrasound flowmeter in man. Eur J Vasc Endovasc Surg 1996; 12:91–96.
7. Louagie YA, Haxhe JP, Jamart J, et al. Doppler flow measurements in coronary artery bypass grafts and early postoperative clinical outcome. J Thorac Cardiovasc Surg 1994; 42:175–181.
8. Canver CC, Cooler SD, Murray EL, Nichols RD, Heisey DM. Clinical importance of measuring coronary graft flows in the revascularized heart: ultrasonic or electromagnetic? J Cardiovasc Surg 1997; 38:211–215.
9. Jaber SF, Koenig SC, BhaskerRao B, VanHimbergen DJ, Spence PA. Can visual assessment of flow waveform morphology detect anastomotic error in off-pump coronary artery bypass grafting? Eur J Cardiothorac Surg 1998; 14:476–479.
10. Mango LJ. Reducing false negatives in clinical practice: the role of neural network technology. Am J Obstet Gynecol 1996; 175(4 pt 2):1114–1119.
11. Smith BM. Interobserver reliability of detecting lumbar intervertebral disc high-intensity zone on magnetic resonance imaging and association of high-intensity zone with pain and anular disruption. Spine 1998; 23(19):2074–2080.
12. Min PU, Griffin BP, Wandervoort PM, Stewart WJ, Fan X, et al. The value of assessing pulmonary venous flow velocity for predicting severity of mitral regurgitation: a quantitative assessment integrating left ventricular function. J Am Soc Echocardiogr 1999; 12(9):736–743.

13. Swenson R. Differential diagnosis: a reasonable clinical approach. Neurol Clin 1999; 17(1):43–63.
14. Koenig SC, VanHimbergen DJ, Jaber SF, Ewert DL, Cerrito P, et al. Spectral analysis of graft flow for anastomotic error detection in off-pump CABG. Eur J Cardiothorac Surg 1999; 16:S83–S87.
15. Warner RM. Spectral Analysis of Time-Series Data. New York, Guilford Press, 1998.
16. Koopmans LH. Kiipmans LH. The Spectral Analysis of Time Series. San Diego, Academic Press.
17. Brigham EO. The Fast Fourier Transform and Its Applications. Upper Saddle River, NJ, Prentice Hall.
18. Haykin SS. Neural Networks: A Comprehensive Foundation. Upper Saddle River, NJ, Prentice Hall.
19. Cerrito PB, Koenig SC, VanHimbergen DJ, Jaber SF, Ewert DL, et al. Neural network pattern recognition analysis of graft flow characteristics improves intraoperative anastomotic error detection in minimally invasive CABG. Eur J Cardiothorac Surg 1999; 16(1):88–93.
20. Pagni S, Salloum E, Storey J, Montgomery W, Cerrito P, et al. Double grafting of the left anterior descending artery: is the distance between the internal mammary artery and supplemental vein graft anastomoses relevant in graft survival? Eur J Cardiothorac Surg 1998; 13(1):36–41.
21. Suma H. Internal thoracic artery and competitive flow. J Thorac Cardiovasc Surg 1991; 102:639–648.
22. Juleff RS, Brow OW, McKain MM, Bendick PJ. The influence of competitive flow on graft patency. J Cardiovasc Surg 1992; 33:415–419.
23. Lust RM, Zeri RS, Spence PA, Chitwood WR. Effect of chronic native flow competition on internal thoracic artery grafts. Ann Thorac Surg 1994; 57:45–50.
24. Mack MJ, Osborne JA, Shennib H. Arterial graft patency in coronary artery bypass grafting: what do we really know? Ann Thorac Surg 1998; 66:1055–1059.

Intraoperative Graft Patency Verification:

Coronary Angiography Versus Transit Time Flow Measurement

Erik Fosse, MD, Per Kristian Hol, MD

Evolution of Treatment of Coronary Disease

Coronary artery revascularization with vein or mammary artery grafts during cardioplegic arrest of the heart has been, for more than 2 decades, the most reliable treatment for coronary artery disease (CAD). Improvements in cardiopulmonary bypass (CPB) technology have reduced perioperative mortality of coronary artery bypass grafting (CABG). Furthermore, surgery has improved long-term outcome when compared to medical treatment.

Since Andreas Grüntzig's publication in 1979,[1] percutaneous coronary angioplasty (PTCA) has become the dominant procedure for coronary revascularization;[2] transluminal treatment of coronary stenosis has been performed mainly by cardiologists and radiologists, while the transthoracic approach has been performed by surgeons. The same phenomenon is found in the managment of congenital heart diseases where transluminal treatment is becoming an important alternative to surgery.[3] The introduction of aortic stents has coupled surgery with catheter techniques. For this reason, integrated operating rooms (ORs) with stationary, high-quality radiological equipment have been used in peripheral vascular surgery, allowing combined radiological and surgical intervention.[4] Until recently, no such "merged rooms" were available in cardiac revascularization.

From: D'Ancona G, Karamanoukian HL, Ricci M, Salerno TA, Bergsland J (eds). *Intraoperative Graft Patency Verification in Cardiac and Vascular Surgery.* © Futura Publishing Company, Armonk, NY, 2001.

In 1996, the Interventional Center at Rikshospitalet (Oslo, Norway) was established with the aim of integrating advanced imaging equipment into the ORs. The first 4 years the Center had 2 ORs, 1 with an open MRI (GE, Signa SP 0.5 Tesla), and 1 with advanced angiographic equipment (Advantix, General Electric Medical Systems, Milwaukee, WI, USA). The department was staffed by surgeons, radiologists, cardiologists, nurses, radiology technicians, and technical engineers.[5] During a 3-year period, 53 coronary operations were performed in the combined suite, together with 33 vascular operations and radiology-guided procedures.[6] During the year 2000, the hospital moved into new facilities and the Interventional Center moved into a new building with 750 square meters of operation facility and 1000 square meters of offices and laboratories. A new hybrid suite was built with new angiography equipment (Siemens, Angiostar, Erlangen, Germany) (Fig. 1). The new center has maintained the open magnetic resonanance imaging (MRI) equipment and presently has a third OR for laparoscopic work and ultrasound-guided procedures.

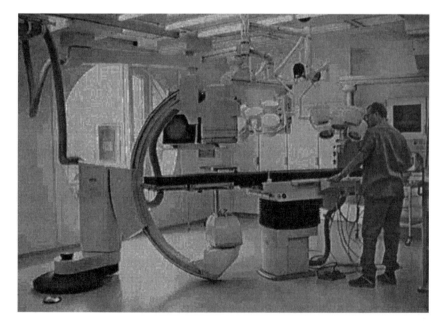

Figure 1. The hybrid suite at the new hospital where advanced angiography equipment (Siemens Angiostar) is installed in a cardiac operating theater. The room is 70 square meters, with a laminar air flow ceiling.

Quality Control of Coronary Grafting

Ever since the beginning of coronary revascularization, the question of estimating graft quality has been addressed. The introduction of beating heart coronary revascularization has increased the need for intraoperative graft and anastomosis quality assessment, because these techniques are more technically demanding. In the past, electromagnetic[7] or Doppler ultrasound flowmeters[8–10] have been used in coronary surgery. Today, transit time flow measurement (TTFM) is the most commonly used technology for intraoperative graft patency verification.[11]

Although transthoracic ultrasound has been used postoperatively to test graft patency of internal mammary artery (IMA) grafts, this method does not give any information about vein grafts.[12] On the contrary, angiography remains the gold standard for postoperative graft patency verification.[13] Due to the possible complications of coronary angiography, this procedure is performed only in patients with recurrent angina or in case of acute myocardial infarction. Intraoperative angiography requires specially designed suites, although portable x-ray equipment has been used.

Development of the Cardiac Procedures at the Interventional Center

After having initially been published by Kolessov[13] in 1967, surgery on the beating heart has recently become a feasible method as documented by Bennetti,[14] Buffolo,[15] and other authors.[16,17] Beating heart cardiac surgery has been performed at the Interventional Center in cooperation with the department of thoracic surgery since 1996. After having successfully operated on 5 animals (pigs), the patient study was started in September 1996. The goal was initially to develop a hybrid procedure where anastomosis of the IMA to the left anterior descending (LAD) artery was performed on the beating heart through a small anterior thoracotomy simultaneously with PTCA and stenting of the other diseased coronary vessels. The first 50 cases were all patients with single-vessel LAD artery disease where the operation was performed through a mini-thoracotomy.

In 10 cases of multivessel disease, a hybrid procedure was performed with surgical revascularization of the LAD through a mini-thoracotomy combined with PTCA of the circumflex and right coronary artery (RCA).[18,19] Today, the hybrid procedure is reserved for special cases because, in the majority of patients, it is possible to simultaneously perform PTCA of the LAD, the RCA, and the circumflex coronary artery. However,

Table 1
Cardiac Procedures in the Combined Suite[21]

LAST	24
Hybrid coronary revascularization	10
Coronary revascularization off-CPB via mid-sternotomy	28
Coronary revascularization on-CPB	19
Closure of sinus-coronary fistula on-CPB	1
Other closed cardiac surgery (off CPB)	1
Transvenous closure of ASD (Amplatzer device)	47
Angioplasty and stent	17
Coronary angiography	18
Animal procedures in the combined suite:	
Closure of ASD	2
Closure of VSD	5
Thoracoscopic/minimally invasive coronary anastomosis	5
Robotic LIMA to LAD anastomosis	5

in re-do cases where the IMA has not been used, the hybrid procedure remains a good option.[20]

From September 1996 to April 2000, 83 patients were operated on in the combined suite. Twenty patients were operated on-CPB and 63 off-CPB. During the same period of time, a total of 17 PTCAs and 47 closures of atrial septal defects by the Amplatzer device (Table 1) were performed in the combined suite. Furthermore, 17 animal procedures were performed in the same suite[21] (Table 1).

Clinical Results and Graft Quality Verification

The clinical outcome in the first 63 patients operated off-CPB was compared to the outcome in the 523 patients treated by conventional cardiac surgery during the same 3-year period. The groups were comparable with respect to gender and age, although after risk stratification using the Higgins and Euro score, the beating heart patients tended to be in a higher risk group. The number of transfusions, intubation time, and incidence of postoperative arrhythmias were all significantly ($P<0.05$) lower in the off-CPB group. Actual mortality was comparable in both groups (1.5%).[23]

Intraoperative angiography was used in the majority of patients operated off-CPB to verify graft patency. Angiography was performed on the table in 56 patients operated off-CPB. All angiographic examinations were performed by 1 radiologist, but evaluated by 3 independent readers. Patency grade was evaluated as described by FitzGibbon.[22] Grafts with good runoff were classified as grade A.

Whenever stenosis reducing the diameter of the grafted artery of more than 50% was present, the graft was classified as grade B. Occluded vessels were categorized as grade O. A total of 77 grafts were evaluated: 51 IMA grafts and 26 vein grafts. Of the 51 IMA grafts, 39 (76%) were completely normal, 10 (20%) had significant lesions, and 2 (4%) were occluded, leading to an on-table grade A+B patency of 96%. The 2 cases with intraoperative occlusion were patients with recanalized, calcified LAD arteries with very small lumen. Revascularization was abandoned due to the condition of the recipient vessel. A total of 26 vein grafts were examined. Of these, 24 were normal, leading to a grade A patency rate of 90%. Two vein grafts (8%) had significant stenoses, and none were occluded. The on-table grade A+B patency rate for vein grafts was thus 100%. A total of 52 patients had follow-up angiography, 24 at 3 months and 28 at 12 months. These 52 patients had a total of 71 grafts: 49 IMA grafts and 22 vein grafts. Of the 49 IMA grafts, 39 (80%) were normal (grade A), 6 (12%) had stenoses (grade B), and 4 (8%) were occluded (grade O). Patency rate with grade A+B was thus 92%. Of the 22 vein grafts, 15 (68%) were normal (grade A), 2 (9%) had significant stenoses (grade B), and 5 (23%) were occluded (grade O), leading to a patency rate A+B of 77%. The overall patency rate (A+B) was 87%.[23]

Transit Time Flow Measurement Findings

At the beginning of our experience with flow measurement, we revised 7 IMA-LAD anastomoses because of abnormal TTFM findings. In 5 other patients, the IMA flow pattern was initially abnormal but returned to normal at the end of the procedure without requiring surgical revision. In these 5 cases, intraoperative angiography revealed grade A anastomoses (Fig. 2 a, b). These unusual findings have led us to compare intraoperative TTFM with intraoperative and follow-up angiography in order to better define the accuracy of TTFM. A total of 67 IMA grafts to the LAD and 57 vein grafts to the circumflex or the RCA were studied. After completion of the anastomosis, flow was measured using the Cardiomed TTFM unit (Medi-Stim, Oslo, Norway). Graft flow rates and waveforms were obtained for each graft. The highest mean flow value was recorded for each graft. For each measurement, the pulsatility index (PI) was calculated in the following way:

$$PI = (systolic\ flow\ 2\ diastolic\ flow)/mean\ flow.$$

At intraoperative angiography, 51 IMAs were grade A, 15 grade B, and 1 grade O. There was no difference in median transit time flow value be-

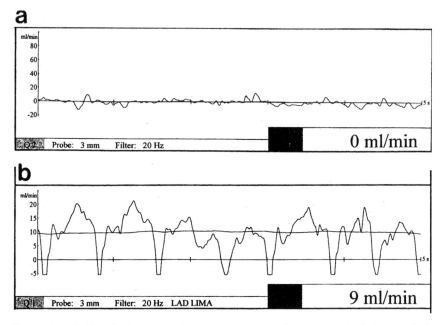

Figure 2. **a, b.** Transit time curve in patient with type A anastomosis, before and after nitroglycerin infusion. The flow was zero in the first measurement, probably due to vessel's spasm.

tween grade A, grade B, and grade O grafts. PI values were also comparable in the 3 groups (Table 2). Similar findings were reported for the vein grafts. In 12 of the 15 patients with grade B grafts, the anastomoses were not revised and patients were restudied after 3 months. At 3-month control, the vessel had remodeled to a grade A graft in 7 patients, while in 5 patients the stenosis persisted. The intraoperative flow and PI did not differ between the vessels that remodeled and the others.[24]

Table 2

Transit Time Flow Measurement and Angiographic Findings in 67 IMA-LAD Grafts

	All Patients	Grade A	Grade B	Grade O
n	67	51	15	1
Transit time flow	22 (3–58)	24 (10–58)	19 (12–39)	5
Pulsatility index	2.3 (1.0–6.5)	2.2 (1.2–6.5)	2.5 (1.0–4.7)	2.3

The anastomoses are graded as A (normal), B (>50% diameter stenosis), and O (occluded). No significant differences were noted in transit time findings of grade A and B grafts.

Discussion

The rapid introduction of new surgical techniques has led to a timely and necessary call for quality control. The TTFM is reliable in detecting anastomoses with a stenosis greater than 90%,[10] but is not reliable when the stenosis is less critical. On the other hand, a less than critical stenosis demonstrated by postoperative angiography may not be hemodynamically relevant because the graft has an ability to remodel over time as already observed by other authors.[25]

A more accurate intraoperative control will lead to better surgical results. Flow measurement equipment is improving, but still the interpretation of intraoperative findings is highly subjective. The integration of imaging equipment into the cardiac OR not only facilitates graft control and assessment, but also allows the development of new procedures erasing the unnatural difference between surgical and cardiological approaches to the treatment of cardiac disease. Team working and eventually the development of new disciplines may assure tailor-made treatment for the individual patient and the disease in contrast to a treatment strategy that is based mainly on the hospital structure. Today the x-ray equipment is still bulky and heavy, making high-quality angiographies and angioplasties during surgery difficult and time-consuming. Portable x-ray machines have been used in coronary revascularization, but they do not give the same quality as standard equipment handled by experts. As eventual postoperative controls are made with stationary equipment, the intraoperative controls should be made with the same quality. However, in the future, image enhancers will be no larger than a small disk, allowing a slim C-bow.

The main problem when using high-precision x-ray equipment is the operative table. The floating table-top required by the radiologists and cardiologists makes tilting facilities complicated. Surgical tables that allow the same freedom of movement as x-ray tables will have to be constructed. Once these problems are solved, integration of advanced angiography into the operating room will probably be common, and intraoperative angiography will be used routinely in most cases.

Future Aspects

New technologies for image acquisitions such as computer tomography (CT), ultrasound, and magnetic resonance imaging (MRI) together with new image-guided therapies have made images very important sources of information in both diagnostics and treatment. In radiology, increasing numbers of examinations are done by MRI. The development of open magnets allowing access to the patient through horizontal or vertical gaps facilitates MRI-guided surgery and intervention. A number of neurosurgical intracranial procedures have been performed in the 0.5 T Sigma Sp magnet (GE, Milwaukee, USA) in several centers including our own.[26]

The open magnets are at present not able to perform good cardiac examinations. In closed magnets, however, visualization of the coronary arteries and grafts is possible. Contrast-enhanced MR angiography for control of coronary stents[27] and coronary grafts has already been demonstrated.[28,29] MRI can also give information on blood flow, velocity, cardiac pump function, myocardial perfusion, and even metabolic processes.[30] New fast magnets will probably be able to present the coronary arteries with the same resolution as angiography today, allowing noninvasive preoperative planning, and intra- and postoperative control of the grafts.

Medical images in digital format are much more suitable for quantitative analysis than the old film and paper format. Computers can be programmed to delimit or define structures or textures of interest for calculation of geometric parameters, localization in space, or other quantitative information. Visualization of such computer-produced information is also important in image-guided therapy. Essential information such as perfusion or blood flow may be emphasized. Digital image processing may also detect unforeseen events that are difficult to spot with some types of displays. Fusion between preoperative and intraoperative images from different modalities could further increase precision and enhance the quality of the image data.[31,32] However, it is very challenging to design appropriate human-machine interfaces without overloading with information. The use of interactive-generated volume data from CT, MRI, 3D ultrasound, or 3D videoscopy in image-guided procedures requires real-time volume rendering and stereo projection techniques. Fusion of images and real-time image processing will most likely be important elements in the treatment of cardiac disease in the future.

References

1. Grüntzig A, Senning Å, Siegenthahl WE. Nonoperative dilatation of coronary artery stenosis: percutaneous transluminal coronary angioplasty. N Engl J Med 1979; 301:61–68.
2. King SB. The development of interventional cardiology. J Am Coll Cardiol 1998; 31:64B–88B.
3. Bjørnstad PG, Masura J, Thaulow E, Smevik B, Michelsen SS, et al. Interventional closure of atrial septal defects with the "Amplatzer" device: first clinical experience. Cardiol in the Young 1997; 7:277–283.
4. Katzen B, Becker GJ, Mascioli CA, Benanti JF, Zemel G, et al. Creation of a modified angiography (endovascular) suite for transluminal endograft placement and combined interventional-surgical procedures. J Vasc Int Radiol 1996; 7:161–167.

5. Lærum F, Borchgrevink HM, Fosse E, Faye-Lund P. The new interventional centre: a multidisciplinary R&D clinic for interventional radiology and minimal access surgery. Comp Methods Progr Biomed 1998; 57:29–34.

6. Fosse E, Lærum F, Røtnes JS. The interventional centre: 30-month experience with a department merging surgery and image-guided intervention. J Min Invasive Ther Technol (in press).

7. Louagie YAG, Haxhe JP, Buche M, Schoevaerdts J-C. Intraoperative electromagnetic flowmeter measurements in coronary artery grafts. J Ann Thorac Surg 1994; 57:357–364.

8. Laustsen J, Pedersen EM, Terp K, Steinbrüchel D, Kure HH, et al. Validation of a new transit time ultrasound flowmeter in man. Eur J Vasc Endovasc Surg 1996; 12:91–96.

9. Cannver CC, Dame NA. Ultrasonic assessment of internal thoracic artery graft in the revascularized heart. Ann Thorac Surg 1994; 58:135–138.

10. Barnea O, Santamore WP. Intraoperative monitoring of IMA flow: what does it mean? Ann Thorac Surg 1997; 63:S12–17.

11. Jaber SF, Koenig SC, BhaskerRao B, VanHimbergen DJ, Spence PA. Can visual assessment of flow waveform morphology detect anastomotic error in off-pump coronary artery bypass grafting? Eur J Cardiothor Surg 1998; 14:476–479.

12. Calafiore AM, Gallina S, Iaco A, Teodori G, Iovino T, et al. Minimally invasive mammary artery Doppler flow velocity evaluation in minimally invasive coronary operations. Ann Thorac Surg 1998; 66:1236–1241.

13. Kolessov VI. Mammary artery-coronary artery anastomosis is a method of treatment for angina pectoris. J Thorac Cardiovasc Surg 1967; 54:535–544.

14. Sani G, Mariani MA, Benetti F, Lisi G, Totaro P, et al. Total arterial myocardial revascularization without cardiopulmonary bypass. Cardiovasc Surg 1996; 4:825–829.

15. Buffolo E, Gerola LR. Coronary artery bypass grafting without cardiopulmonary bypass through sternotomy and minimally invasive procedures. Int J Cardiol 1997; 62(suppl):89–93.

16. Bergsland J, Schmid S, Yanulecvich J, Hasnain S, Lajos TZ, et al. Coronary artery bypass grafting (CABG) without cardiopulmonary bypass (CPB): a strategy for improving results in surgical revascularization. Heart Surg Forum 1998; 1:107–110.

17. Loop FD, Lytle BW, Cosgrove DM, Stewart RW, Goormastic M, et al. Influence of the internal mammary artery graft on 10-year survival and other cardiac events. N Engl J Med 1986; 314:1–6.

18. Barstad RM, Fosse E, Vatne K, Andersen K, Tønnessen TI, et al. Intraoperative evaluation of bypass anastomosis during MIDCAB: the value of intraoperative coronary angiography. Ann Thorac Surg 1997; 64:1835–1839.

19. Barstad RM, Fosse E, Geiran OR, Simonsen S, Vatne K, et al. Minimally invasive direct coronary artery bypass grafting without cardiopulmonary bypass in combination with intraoperative percutaneous transluminal coronary angioplasty for palliative coronary revascularization in a heart-transplant recipient. J Heart Lung Transplant 1998; 17:629–634.

20. Angelini GD, Wilde P, Salerno TA, Bosco G, Calafiore AM. Integrated left anterior small thoracotomy and angioplasty for multivessel coronary artery revascularization. Lancet 1996; 347:757–758.

21. Fosse E, Samseth E, Elle OJ, Hol PK, Bjørnstad P, et al. Integrating Image Guidance into the Cardiac OR. MITAT 2000.

22. FitzGibbon GM, Burton JR, Leach AJ. Coronary bypass graft fate: angiographic grading of 1400 consecutive grafts early after operation and of 1132 after one year. Circulation 1978; 57:1070–1074.
23. Hol PK, Fosse E, Svennevig JL, Geiran O, Lundblad R, et al. Off-pump coronary artery bypass surgery with angiographic follow-up. Manuscript in preparation.
24. Hol PK, Fosse E, Mørk BE, Lundblad R, Rein KA, et al. Graft control by transit time flow measurement and intraoperative angiography in coronary bypass surgery. Manuscript in preparation.
25. Calafiore AM, Di Giammarco G. Mid-term results after minimally invasive coronary surgery (the last operation). J Thorac Cardiovasc Surg 1998; 115:763–771.
26. Jolesz FA. MRI-guided interventions. The Coolidge 1994; 2:1–15.
27. De Cobelli F, Cappio S, Vanzulli A, Del Maschio A. MRI assessment of coronary stents. Rays 1999; 1924:140–148.
28. Brenner P, Wintersperger B, von Smekal A, Agirov V, Bohm D, et al. Detection of coronary artery bypass graft patency by contrast-enhanced magnetic resonance angiography. Eur J Cardiothorac Surg 1999; 1915:389–393.
29. Boehm DH, Wintersperger BJ, Reichenspurner H, Gulbins H, Detter C, et al. Contrast-enhanced magnetic resonance angiography for control of minimally invasive coronary artery bypass conduits. Heart Surg Forum 1999; 2:222–225.
30. Smith H-J. Cardiac MR imaging. Acta Radiologica 1999; 40:1–22.
31. Meyer CR, Boes JL, Kim B, Bland PH, Zasadny KR, et al. Demonstration of accuracy and clinical versatility of mutual information for automatic multimodality image fusion using affine and thin-plate spline-warped geometric deformations. Med Image Anal 1997; 1:195–206.
32. Alpert NM, Berdichevsky D, Levin Z, Morris ED, Fischman AJ. Improved methods for image registration. Neuroimage 1996; 3:10–18.

10

Intraoperative Flow Measurements:

Predictive Value for Postoperative Angiographic Follow-Up

Yves A.G. Louagie, MD, PhD,
Carlos E. Brockmann, MD, O. Gurné, MD, PhD,
Jacques Jamart, MD

Introduction

The predictive value of intraoperative measurements of hemodynamic parameters, for long-term coronary bypass graft patency, remains a matter of controversy. Indeed, Walker,[1] Grondin,[2] Moran,[3] and Björk[4] demonstrated that flow in the graft, as measured during surgery, was an important determinant of later patency. By contrast, the mean flow measured before chest closure was found to have no predictive value by Balderman[5] and de Rijbel.[6] These studies were completed between 1970 to 1980 and used electromagnetic flow measurements made in saphenous vein bypass grafts.[1–3,5,6] However, similar investigations were never carried out for arterial grafts. Since the introduction of the electromagnetic flowmeter, the significance of these initial observations was clearly limited because they used methods restricted to the measurement of mean flow and the analysis of phasic flow patterns.

There is thus a need to thoroughly assess the hemodynamic features

From: D'Ancona G, Karamanoukian HL, Ricci M, Salerno TA, Bergsland J (eds). *Intraoperative Graft Patency Verification in Cardiac and Vascular Surgery.* © Futura Publishing Company, Armonk, NY, 2001.

of arterial and saphenous vein bypass grafts in relation to their later patency. Several questions have to be answered:

1. Can intraoperative flow measurements predict later graft patency?
2. Can intraoperative flow measurements predict later graft stenosis?
3. Which hemodynamic parameter is the best predictor?
4. Do hemodynamic parameters retain their potential predictive value if patient-related variables are taken into account?

Dual-Beam Doppler Flowmeter

Description of Flowmeter Methodology

Data were obtained using a pulsed Doppler flowmeter adapted to the assessment of both arterial and venous coronary bypass grafts.[7–9] An 8-MHz pulsed-wave Doppler ultrasound flowmeter (OPDOP 130, Scimed, Bristol, UK) was used. The system uses an annular array transducer that is capable of transmitting and receiving 2 concentric ultrasound beams (Fig.

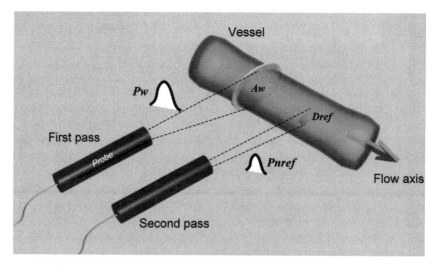

Figure 1. Pulsed wave Doppler placement with the 2 concentric Doppler beams directed on the vessel. The system uses an annular array transducer that is capable of transmitting and receiving 2 concentric ultrasound beams. One is a wide beam (Aw) in which the sample volume receives Doppler information from the total cross-sectional area of the vessel (first pass). The other is a narrow beam (Dref) in which the sample volume receives Doppler information from a small defined area within the vessel lumen (second pass). Pw is the total Doppler power from the insonated vessel diameter, and Pnref is the power from the known sample volume size.

1). The system has 2 receiver gates: one that receives Doppler information from the entire diameter of the vessel (Aw), and a smaller gate of known size (Dref), corresponding mostly to half the clip size that receives information from the middle of the vessel. By comparing the Doppler power received by the larger gate with that of the smaller gate, the diameter of the vessel can be calculated from the equation:

$$D = [Pw/Pnref] \times Dref$$

where Pw is the total Doppler power received from the insonated vessel diameter and Pnref is the power from the smaller sample of known volume. The mean flow velocity is obtained from the mean Doppler shift frequency observed at the larger gate. This velocity is calculated based on the Doppler equation:

$$Fd = 2 \cdot f \cdot (v/c) \cdot \cos \theta$$

where Fd is the transmit frequency, f is the ultrasonic carrier frequency, v is the velocity, c equals 1600 m/sec, and cos θ equals 0.5 (cos 60°). The ultimate flow is then defined by:

$$Q = k \cdot Fd \cdot [Pw/Pnref) \cdot Dref]^2 \cdot \pi/4$$

Flow measurements were obtained by constraining the vessel in a plastic cuff made of 2 halves clipped around it. A range of cuffs, from 3 to 12 mm diameter in 1-mm steps, is available to provide satisfactory adaptation to the size of the vessel. The cuffs normally used had a diameter of 4 mm (mean 4.0 ± 0.0 mm; range 3–6 mm for internal thoracic artery grafts, and a mean of 4.4 ± 0.1 mm; range 3–7 mm for saphenous vein grafts, P=0.002). The ultrasound pencil probe is slotted into the cuff and acoustically coupled to the vessel using a small amount of sterile gel. Care must be taken to avoid large air bubbles in the coupling gel that could severely damp the signal. The probe to the vessel angle is fixed at 60°. Sharp dissection is not necessary to measure flow in the internal thoracic artery, since the cuff can easily be applied around the artery in an area where it is level with the anterior aspect of the musculofascial pedicle. An intraoperative flow measurement is illustrated in Figure 2, and a velocity profile is depicted in Figure 3.

The flow in the grafts was measured on bypass, immediately after completion of the proximal anastomoses, while the patient was rewarmed to 36°C. Recording sites were in the proximal vein graft segment, the mid-portion of the internal thoracic artery pedicle, or the internal epigastric artery. In the case of sequential bypass grafts, blood flow velocities were measured in

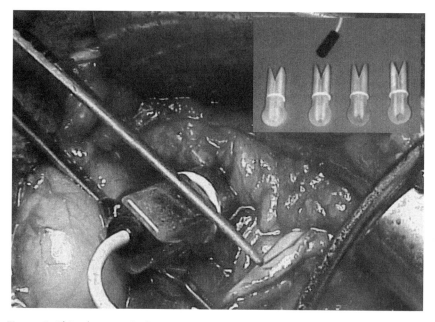

Figure 2. This photograph depicts intraoperative flow measurement in a gastroepiploic artery graft. The insert shows the Doppler probe and various clip sizes.

the region proximal to the side-to-side anastomosis. For the gastroepiploic artery, the surrounding fat was incised at a level situated 2 to 3 cm distal from the origin of the gastroduodenal artery. Our experience with flow measurements in the gastroepiploic artery have been described previously.[10,11]

Validation Studies

A detailed description and validation of the method used has been published.[9] For the internal thoracic artery, results obtained with Doppler ultrasound were first correlated with measures attained simultaneously on the same graft, by timed-volume collection of blood when the distal graft was open. This represents the absolute value (Fig. 4). There was a satisfactory correlation between both measurements (r=0.86, P<0.0001, n=32) with a slight flow overestimation using Doppler ultrasound (Doppler flow = 17.6 + 0.97 flow by volume collection).

The method was further validated for the saphenous vein graft in an artificial circuit with the flow measured by dual-beam Doppler (Fig. 4). A Doppler probe was placed on a saphenous vein, 3.0 mm in internal diameter. The vessel was connected to a roller pump, and flow (range 20 to 100

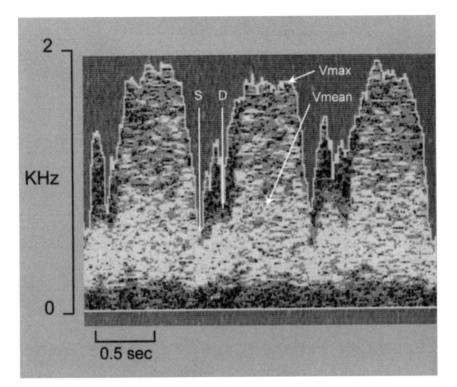

Figure 3. Typical velocity pattern of 3 cardiac cycles in a grafted left internal thoracic artery. S = onset of systole; D = onset of diastole; V–max = maximal velocity; V–mean = mean velocity.

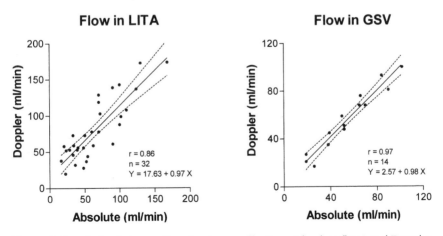

Figure 4. Correlation between timed-volume collections (absolute flow) and Doppler flow measurements performed in situ in a left internal thoracic artery (LITA) and in vitro in a greater saphenous vein (GSV). See text for further information. (Adapted from ref.[9] with permission.)

mL/min) was assessed by timed-volume collection. The fluid used was whole citrate-treated human blood (hemoglobin content 14.9 g/100 mL; hematocrit 44.7%). Measurements of flow and timed-volume collection were performed at multiple flow rates. There was an excellent correlation between both techniques of flow measurement (r=0.97, P<0.001, n=14).

Hemodynamic Parameters

The parameters determined by pulsed Doppler were flow (mL/min), velocity (cm/sec), and internal diameter (mm) of the vessel. Furthermore, the total resistance of the graft and coronary bed was calculated using the OPDOP 130 software from the mean radial artery pressure, divided by mean flow measured after completion of the coronary anastomoses, and is expressed in peripheral resistance units (PRU). A pulsatility index (PI) was calculated to describe the shape of the curves. This is a dimensionless variable, independent of probe-to-vessel angle. This variable is defined as follows:

$$PI = (Fmax - Fmin)/Fmean$$

where Fmax is the maximum frequency, Fmin is the minimum frequency, and Fmean is the mean frequency. In addition, the pulsed Doppler flowmeter can be connected to a real-time spectrum analyzer (Dopstation, Scimed, Bristol, UK), and the Doppler audio signals processed by the spectrum analyzer by means of online fast Fourier transformation. In this way, directional spectral information, including the maximum and mean frequency traces, can be displayed in real-time (Fig. 3).

Velocity Patterns

Flow velocity patterns were assessed using a classification established by Balderman et al.,[5] who assigned a qualitative grade to each phasic flow curve on a scale of 1 to 4. Grade 1 is characterized by a flow with rapid and smooth acceleration and deceleration in the diastolic phase. Grade 2 represents mildly prolonged acceleration and deceleration, with some irregularities. Grade 3 represents moderately prolonged acceleration and deceleration with moderate tracing irregularities, and less distinction between diastolic and systolic flow tracing irregularities. Grade 4 represents poor acceleration and deceleration of flow with marked irregularities in the tracings, and poor distinction between diastolic and systolic flow components. Examples of typical velocity profiles are shown in Figure 5.

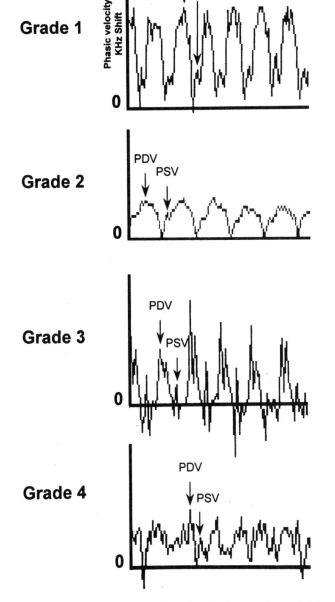

Figure 5. Examples of phasic velocity profiles classified according to Balderman[5] (see text for further information). PDV and PSV indicate peak diastolic and peak systolic velocity, respectively.

Study Design

Patient Population

Assessment of coronary bypass grafts by a pulsed Doppler flowmeter was carried out in 894 consecutive patients, operated on from November 1989 to October 1996 by the same surgeon (Y.L.).[12] Among these patients, 85 (9.5%) underwent an angiographic control required by the suspected recurrence of angina (n=50, 59%) or as part of a prospective study undertaken to document graft status (n=35, 41%). These 85 patients, with both technically adequate intraoperative graft flow assessment and repeat postoperative angiography, were included in the present study. Intraoperative Doppler measurements and selective graft injection at control angiography were obtained for 214 bypasses in 238 implanted grafts (90%).

The mean age at operation was 61.2 ± 1.0 years. There were 71 men and 14 women. The indications for bypass grafting included unstable angina in 30 patients (35.3%) and angina after recent (< 6 weeks) myocardial infarction in 11 patients (12.9%). The extent of coronary artery disease at angiography was as follows: left main disease (isolated or associated), 10 patients; 1-vessel disease, 2 patients; 2-vessel disease, 30 patients; and 3-vessel disease, 50 patients. The left ventricular ejection fraction was obtained angiographically in 45 patients and averaged 0.62 ± 0.02. It was measured by radioisotope in less favorable cases in 14 patients and averaged 0.45 ± 0.03.

Repeat catheterization was performed within 1 month of surgery in 16 patients and later (median 17 months: range 1 to 83 months) in 69 patients. Grafts were angiographically classified as intact, meaning widely patent with no perceptible narrowing or stenosis, or occluded. Nonoccluded grafts, including stenotic grafts, were classified as patent. The stenotic category included grafts with subcritical stenoses (including new angiographic irregularities), as well as grafts that were severely stenotic and hemodynamically compromised. The entire length of the grafts and the anastomoses were considered. If multiple stenoses were present, the graft was classified according to the most severe narrowing.

Surgical Techniques

All distal anastomoses were performed during a single interval of aortic cross-clamping, and the aortic anastomoses were carried out with tangential aortic cross-clamping while the heart was kept in the empty beating state. The luminal diameter of the recipient coronary arteries was measured with malleable probes in 0.5-mm gradations. In all, 245 distal anastomoses were constructed (2.9 per patient; range 1 to 4). One hundred and five anastomoses (43%) were completed with arterial grafts, whereas 140 anastomoses (57%) were performed with venous grafts. Sixty-nine patients (81%) underwent the implantation of a single internal thoracic artery and 12 patients (14%) had bilateral internal thoracic artery grafting. Sequential bypass grafting was performed in 7 patients. An epigastric artery was implanted in 5 patients and a gastroepiploic artery was grafted to the posterior descending artery in 6 patients. Six patients had re-do procedures.

Data Analysis

Perioperative data, including hemodynamic measurements for the grafts, were collected and entered prospectively into a clinical research database. Values were presented as mean ± standard error of the mean. Statistical analysis was performed with use of the SPSS software package (SPSS Inc., Chicago, IL), unless otherwise specified. Categorical clinical data were compared between 2 populations by chi-square tests. Intergroup comparisons (intact graft, stenosis, occlusion) were performed by Kruskal-Wallis exact (or Monte Carlo) permutation tests for categorical variables and Jonckheere-Tepstra exact permutation tests for ordered variables. Both of these tests were performed using StatXact software (Cytel Software Corporation, Cambridge, MA). Graft hemodynamic parameters, expressed as continuous variables, were compared between the aforementioned 3 groups by 1-way analysis of variance followed by Scheffé tests for 2 × 2 comparisons.

Graft patency curves were constructed by the Kaplan-Meier method, and compared by a log-rank test, assuming independence of the grafts in the same patient.

Graft patency rates were compared by regression analysis of repeated measures, using generalized estimating equations as described by Liang and Zeger,[13] the occlusion of the graft being considered as the dependent variable. The latter analysis allowed us to take into account patient-related and graft-related variables simultaneously, and was performed using the RMGEE program.[14] Backward selection with a $P<0.05$ limit was used. In the first analysis, only graft hemodynamic data were considered. These variables included flow, velocity, resistance, PI, and internal diameter. Both graft- and patient-specific characteristics were included in a second analysis.

Receiver-operator-characteristic (ROC) curves were used to validate the predictive value of the subset of variables that correlated the best with later patency. ROC curves were constructed by means of maximum likelihood estimation under the binormal model,[15] using the LABROC1 program (C.E. Metz, University of Chicago, Chicago, IL).

Study Limitations

This study has several limitations. First, it must be emphasized that our series is selected, since the majority of our patients were studied for recurrent symptoms. Thus, our conclusions may not necessarily be applied generally to all patients following coronary revascularization. However, for the purpose of this study, such selection constitutes an advantage. Second, measurements taken at operation may not truly reflect the capacity of the graft to carry blood flow, because the heart may not have fully recovered from the consequences of ischemic arrest. However, consecutive flow measurements, made from aortic unclamping until the end of the procedure, show that the highest flow was obtained immediately after weaning from cardiopulmonary bypass.[16] Furthermore, induction of hyperemia by papaverine injection directly into the graft did not significantly improve the predictive value of previous flow studies.[2,3] Third, analysis of the results poses an important methodological problem because the characteristics of any one patient (i.e., age, diabetes, hypercholesterolemia) are correlated with the various features of several bypass grafts and recipient arteries (i.e., flow, coronary diameter). Indeed, for the purpose of the analysis, each bypass graft was considered individually. Thus, patient-related factors such as diabetes will influence the fate of all the grafts of a given patient and thus will need to be taken into account several times (equivalent to the amount of distal anastomoses) in logistic regression analysis. Therefore, the generalized estimating equation approach, which takes into account and corrects the latter bias, was preferred to the more usual multiple regression analysis. Conversely, to carry out Kaplan-Meier analysis, we had to assume that the fates of all grafts were independent, although clusters of grafts from the same patient were obviously exposed to a unique set of risk factors. Finally, the present study is limited to early and mid-term angiographic follow-up. Although the operation-to-catheterization interval was longer than in the majority of the previous studies, it rarely exceeded 5 years. On the other hand, determinants of early graft closure differ from the determinants of late graft closure.[17,18] Thus, after a longer follow-up duration, the marked influence of intraoperative hemodynamic measurements may be overshadowed by risk factors for atherosclerosis and by the nature of the bypass conduits.

Factors Influencing Mid-Term Graft Patency

The overall graft patency rate was 88.3%. Among patients undergoing angiographic evaluation as part of a systematic graft control program, the patency rate was 93.4%. Not surprisingly, the patency rate dropped to 84.6% when angiography was required because of a recurrence of symptoms (P=0.035).

Nature of the Bypass Conduit

The nature of the graft had a marked influence on patency, since the overall difference between grafts was significant (P=0.008). The arterial grafts had a global patency rate of 94% (84/89), contrasting with a patency rate of 84% (105/125) for saphenous vein bypass grafts (P=0.020). Figure 6 demonstrates the superior patency rate of the arterial grafts over the saphenous vein grafts. In addition, left internal thoracic artery grafts had better patency rates than did those for the right internal thoracic artery, the

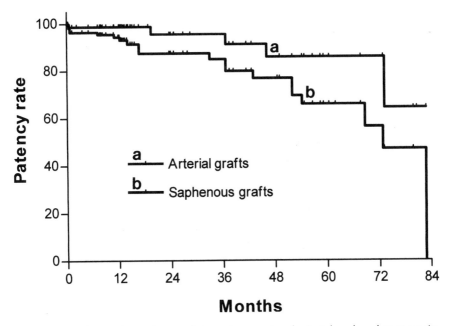

Figure 6. Kaplan-Meier estimate of the patency rate of arterial and saphenous vein coronary bypass grafts. The comparison of graft patency curves by a log-rank test demonstrated a significant difference (P=0.013).

internal epigastric artery, or the saphenous vein. Nevertheless, these data need to be interpreted cautiously since a given bypass graft is often associated with a specific runoff bed. For example, the left internal thoracic artery was in the vast majority of cases grafted to the widest runoff bed, which is the left anterior descending artery.

Morphological Features of the Host Vessels

The degree of coronary stenosis as determined at the preoperative angiography did not influence graft patency. By contrast, the size of the artery, as measured with intra-arterial probes at the site of anastomosis, markedly influenced postoperative patency, principally in arteries under a 1.5-mm internal diameter ($P<0.001$). Indeed, the occlusion rate reached 62% in arteries of less than 1-mm internal diameter and 38% in arteries ranging from 1 to 1.4 mm internal diameter (Fig. 7). The quality of the grafted coronary artery was also of significance ($P=0.016$), since heavily calcified arteries and the presence of atheromatous plaques were associated with higher occlusion rates. Finally, the location of the target coro-

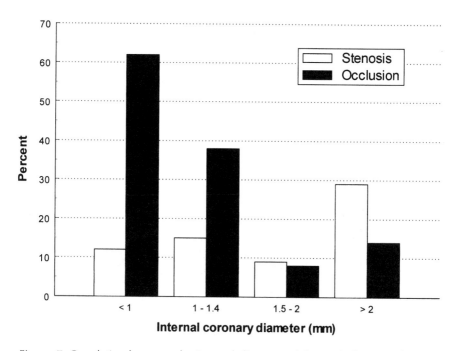

Figure 7. Correlation between the internal diameter of the grafted coronary artery and the incidence of late occlusion and stenosis.

nary artery affected outcome. The grafts implanted onto the left anterior descending artery had the highest patency rate.

Hemodynamic Assessment of Grafts

The mean flow measured intraoperatively in 168 intact grafts at angiographic follow-up was 60 ± 3 mL/min (range 9 to 230 mL/min), and the resistance was 1.8 ± 0.1 PRU (range 0.3 to 9.0 PRU) (Table 1). By contrast, mean intraoperative flow was only 36 ± 5 mL/min (range 2 to 107 mL/min), and resistance reached 5.9 ± 2.0 PRU (range 0.6 to 46.0 PRU) in 25 grafts found occluded at angiographic evaluation. By univariate analysis, reduced flow, reduced velocity, increased resistance, and PI were all significantly associated with a higher occlusion rate. The correlation between resistance and graft status at control angiography is shown in Figure 8. A wide dispersion of the resistance values was observed in the cases of occlusion. The combined influence of 2 hemodynamic parameters on graft patency was tested and expressed in a 3-dimensional graph, as shown in Figure 9, for the interaction between reduced flow and increased resistance. However, multivariate analysis performed on graft-related hemodynamic variables selected increased resistance as the only independent variable that correlated with postoperative occlusion (P=0.011).

In 3 groups, arbitrarily separated according to a range of resistance values, the patency rate was 96 ± 4% at 5 years for the group with a resis-

Table 1
Correlation Between Intraoperative Graft Hemodynamic Assessment and Postoperative Patency

| | Angiographic Outcome | | | | P |
Graft Hemodynamics	Intact	Stenosis	Occlusion	Overall	Value*
Flow (mL/min)	60 ± 3[†]	49 ± 6	36 ± 5[†]	56 ± 3	0.011
Velocity (cm/s)	19 ± 1[†]	17 ± 2	11 ± 2[†]	18 ± 1	0.002
Resistance (PRU)	1.8 ± 0.1[¶]	2.3 ± 0.6[¶]	5.9 ± 2.0[¶]	2.3 ± 0.3	0.000
Mean pressure (mm Hg)	75 ± 1	76 ± 2	79 ± 2	75 ± 1	0.201
Pulsatility index	2.5 ± 0.2[¶]	2.4 ± 0.4[¶]	8.1 ± 3.0[¶]	3.1 ± 0.4	0.000
Internal diameter (mm)	2.6 ± 0.1	2.6 ± 0.1	2.7 ± 0.1	2.6 ± 0.0	0.897

Adapted from ref.[12], with permission.
Values are expressed as mean ± SEM.
PRU = peripheral resistance units.
* Analysis of variance.
Significant (P<0.05) intergroup differences by Scheffe test.
† Intact versus occlusion.
¶ Intact versus occlusion and stenosis versus occlusion.

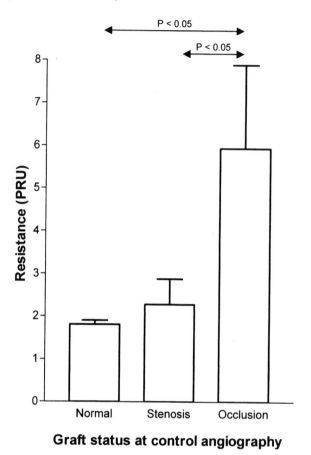

Figure 8. Correlation between resistance as measured intraoperatively and graft status at control angiography. Error bars indicate standard errors of the mean. PRU = peripheral resistance units.

tance < 1 PRU, 74 ± 7% for the group with a resistance ranging from 1 to 3 PRU, and 43 ± 15% for the group with a resistance ≥3 PRU (Fig. 10).

Stenoses were characterized by their grade and locality. Twenty-one grafts were stenosed to a degree that ranged from 30% to 90% (average, 66.4 ± 4.9%). The stenosis was proximal in 6 saphenous vein grafts, and anastomotic in 5 internal thoracic artery grafts and 4 saphenous vein grafts. In addition, a stenosis was situated in the middle part of a saphenous vein graft whereas multiple stenoses were diffusely distributed in 2 other saphenous vein grafts. Three arterial grafts (2 internal thoracic arteries and 1 epigastric artery) had a string appearance. Given the variability of these features, we were not able to draw any firm conclusions re-

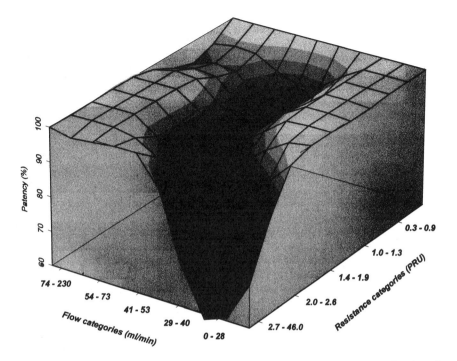

Figure 9. Three-dimensional representation of the combined influence of reduced flow (X-axis) and increased resistance (Y-axis) on graft patency (Z-axis). For the purpose of the graph, flow and resistance values are presented as percentile categories.

garding the predictive value of any of the graft- or patient-related parameters for late stenosis.

Velocity Curve Patterns

The correlation between the velocity patterns classified according to Balderman and associates[5] and the graft occlusion rate is shown in Figure 11. The grade 1 curves were the easiest to identify, whereas grades 3 and 4 curves were more difficult to differentiate. In grafts with grade 1 patterns, the patency rate was 98%, whereas grafts with grades 2 to 4 patterns had an overall patency rate of 84% (P=0.008). This represents a sensitivity of 96% and a specificity of only 31%. Indeed, the differentiation between the systolic and diastolic phases of the flow pattern is impeded in bypasses to the right coronary system because flow is antegrade throughout the pulse cycle, reflecting the lower intramural systolic compressive forces of the right ventricle. By contrast, in grafts that predominantly supply the left ventricle, the flow pattern is characterized by a short systolic peak, followed by a well-delimited and predominantly

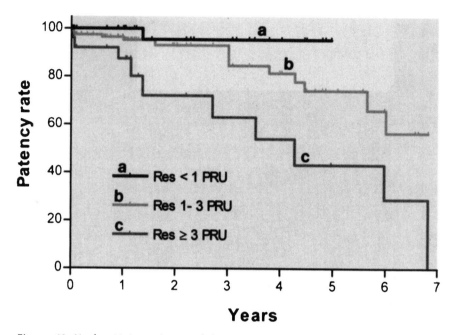

Figure 10. Kaplan-Meier estimate of the patency rate according to the resistance measured intraoperatively. The comparison of graft patency curves by a log-rank test demonstrated a significant difference (P=0.0019).

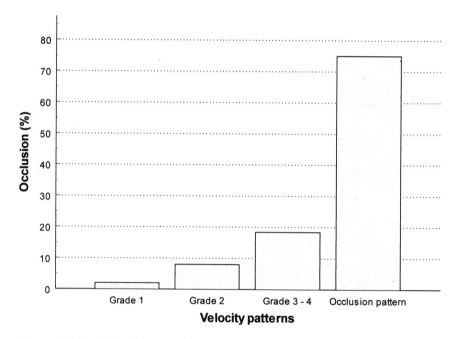

Figure 11. Correlation between the velocity patterns and the incidence of graft occlusion.

diastolic flow of longer duration. Therefore, when the grafts are separated according to their runoff bed into left-system grafts (supplying left anterior descending, diagonal, or marginal arteries) and right-system grafts (supplying right coronary or posterior descending arteries), only the velocity profiles of the left-system grafts are discriminative for postoperative graft patency (P< 0.001).

Finally, a high-resistance velocity pattern, suggestive of outflow obstruction, was evidenced in 4 grafts. The abnormal waveform configuration was characterized by sharp spikes and well-detached phasic flow patterns in systole and diastole. All of these grafts were found to be occluded or stenosed.

Multivariate Analysis of Factors Likely to Influence Patency

Patient- and graft-specific variables simultaneously assessed by generalized estimating equations are listed in Table 2. Three independent variables were associated with a reduced patency rate: increased resistance as measured in the graft (P=0.012); increasing interval of control angiography (P=0.006); and preoperative cardiogenic shock (P=0.040). The nature of the bypass conduit was not selected by the multivariate analysis as an independent variable influencing graft outcome.

Constructing ROC curves (Fig. 12) further validated the predictive value of the subset of 3 variables, in which the combinations of risk factors were reported as observed points. These curves plot the sensitivity (i.e., the proportion of occluded grafts correctly predicted) versus specificity (i.e., the proportion of erroneous classification of graft occlusion) for every possible value of the function. The area under the ROC curve is thus a global measure of the accuracy of the classification rule, whatever threshold is chosen. The area under the ROC curve was 0.766 ± 0.054. The ROC curve can vary from 0.5 (no discrimination) to 1.0 (perfect discrimination).

Discussion

A striking influence of the nature of the bypass conduit on patency was shown by univariate analysis: the patency rate of arterial grafts was by far superior to venous grafts. This has been a well-established concept since the works of Lytle[18] and Zeff.[19] However, the nature of the bypass conduit was not selected in the multivariate analysis as an independent variable influencing graft outcome, the resistance of the runoff bed being dominant. This can be explained by the fact that our study involves a majority of mid-term (< 5 years interval) angiographic controls. Moreover,

Table 2

Variables Used in the Multivariate Analysis

Independent variables
Patient specific
  Age (years)
  Gender (male or female)
  Systemic hypertension (1 or 0)
  Diabetes mellitus (1 or 0)
  Smoking habits (1 or 0)
  Lipid abnormalities (1 or 0)
  Renal dysfunction (1 or 0)
  Obesity (1 or 0)
  Chronic obstructive lung disease (1 or 0)
  History of remote myocardial infarction ($\geq$6 weeks) (1 or 0)
  History of recent myocardial infarction (<6 weeks) (1 or 0)
  Angina class (1 to 4)
  Transfer from intensive care unit (1 or 0)
  Cardiogenic shock (1 or 0)
  Intra-aortic balloon counterpulsation (1 or 0)
  Intravenous nitrates (1 or 0)
  Elective, urgent, or emergency procedure (1 to 3)
  Interval of control angiography (months)
Graft-host vessel specific
Host vessel features
  Coronary artery territory grafted (1 to 9)
  Proximal stenosis (50 to 100%)
  Internal diameter of coronary artery (mm)
  Morphologic features of coronary artery (1 to 5)*
Graft features
  Nature of bypass conduit (1 to 4)**
  Flow (mL/min)
  Velocity (cm/s)
  Resistance (mm Hg/mL/min^{-1})
  Pulsatility index (index)
  Internal diameter of graft (mm)
Dependent variable
Graft occluded (1 or 0)

Adapted from ref.[12] with permission.
* 1 = normal; 2 = atheromatous plaque at the anastomosis; 3 = diffusely atheromatous; 4 = very atheromatous; 5 = need for endarterectomy.
** 1 = internal thoracic artery; 2 = epigastric artery; 3 = gastroepiploic artery; 4 = saphenous vein.

the attrition rate of vein grafts starts to exceed that of mammary artery grafts markedly from 5 years after the operation.[18] The same observations were made by van der Meer et al.,[20] who demonstrated the absence of difference in adjusted risk of 1-year occlusion rates between internal thoracic artery grafts and vein grafts. By contrast, the location of the distal anasto-

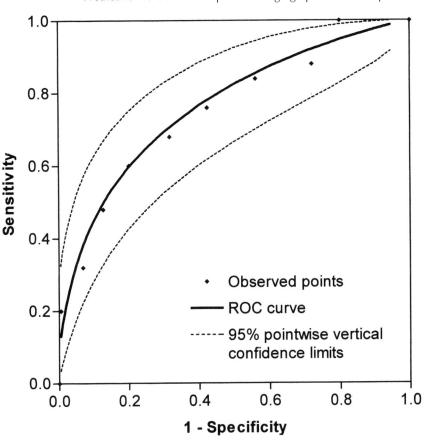

Figure 12. Receiver-operative characteristics (ROC) curve assessing the predictive value for graft occlusion of the set of variables evidenced by the multivariate analysis. The area under the curve is 0.766 ± 0.054.

mosis and the lumen diameter of the grafted coronary artery were shown to be significant predictors of occlusion.

Regarding the morphological features of the recipient vessels, there was no significant difference in the patency rate with varying degrees of coronary arterial stenosis or total occlusion. This corroborates the findings of Crosby et al.,[21] who demonstrated that the patency rate of saphenous vein grafts was not significantly lower, even in vessels with less than 60% stenosis, and even though competitive flow appears to predispose to graft occlusion. Likewise, Manninen et al.[22] showed that the patency of arterial graft anastomoses was independent of the degree of the stenosis bypassed. Nevertheless, it was demonstrated for arterial grafts[23–25] that midterm patency rate depends on flow through the native coronary artery, a graft occlusion, or a thinning down phenomenon associated with mild coronary stenosis at initial angiography.

By contrast, the coronary artery diameter, measured at the level of the anastomosis, was a good predictor of graft patency, since the occlusion rate increased strikingly in coronary vessels with an internal diameter inferior to 1.5 mm. Indeed, a larger coronary artery is not only easier to graft, but its distal bed is also better developed, as demonstrated by the finding that a maximally dilated coronary artery luminal cross-sectional area is linearly related to the volume of muscle it perfuses.[26]

Several intraoperative hemodynamic parameters were found associated with postoperative graft occlusion by univariate analysis: reduced flow, reduced velocity, increased resistance, and increased PI. By multivariate analysis, increased resistance was the only significant predictor among flow-derived data. Supporting this, Moran and associates[3] measured a high resistance, ranging from 2.5 to 8.0 PRU, in 4 instances of graft occlusion.

A combination of patient- and graft-specific parameters was assessed by multivariate analysis. Again, increased resistance was demonstrated to have a strong effect on later graft patency. The influence of increased intervals of the control angiography from the initial procedure is obvious, since the risk of graft occlusion increases with time, which confirms the findings of previous studies.[18]

Although a reasonably satisfactory predictive value could be attributed to intraoperative graft hemodynamic assessment regarding the risk of later occlusion, these measurements were useless to predict stenosis. Intraoperative hemodynamic parameters did not differ between intact and stenosed grafts. Indeed, stenosis development is related to scar tissue or to degeneration of a graft, a phenomenon that cannot be detected at the procedure and is predominantly patient-related. In addition, the localization and the degree of stenosis are highly variable.

Furthermore, the immediate detection of mild stenoses is very difficult with the available Doppler flowmeters. Indeed, Jaber and associates[27] demonstrated that visual assessment of flow waveform morphology can help to detect nearly occluded (>90% stenosis) anastomoses intraoperatively, but is unreliable for assessing intermediate stenosis. Differences in mean graft flow are detectable in anastomoses with severe stenosis (>75%) but not in anastomoses with mild (<25%) to moderately severe (<75%) stenosis.[28] Only sophisticated methods such as spectral analysis of graft flow waveforms may allow the detection of lesser degrees of anastomotic stenosis.[29] Finally, flow in the recipient coronary artery can compete with flow in the graft and obscure the diagnosis of mild stenosis. Nevertheless, D'Ancona and associates[30] suppressed that limitation of the method by snaring the proximal coronary artery to enhance the graft specificity of the flow measurement.

Thus, since available flow measurement techniques are unable to detect mild stenoses, they are certainly inaccurate for predicting their later progression. Fortunately, the prediction of late stenosis development is much less crucial than the prediction of late graft occlusion. Lytle[31] demonstrated that patients with circumflex or right coronary artery vein graft stenosis had a survival equivalent to that of their control group. By contrast, late stenoses in saphenous vein grafts to the left anterior descending coronary artery predicted high rates of both death and cardiac events and were an indication for operation. However, saphenous veins are only exceptionally used as conduits to bypass that territory today.

This study has several clinical implications. Intraoperative hemodynamic graft assessment and, particularly, resistance measured in the grafts may provide a good prognostic index and be of value in the selection of patients for postoperative angiographic evaluation. In addition, graft resistance, as determined at the initial operation, may represent a valuable guide to the possible success of repeat surgery, should this become necessary. Arterial conduits had a superior patency rate than saphenous vein grafts. However, the nature of the conduit, including patient-specific parameters such as gender, smoking habits, hypertension, lipid abnormalities, or diabetes, had no bearing on mid-term graft patency by multivariate analysis.

Summary

The predictive value for early and mid-term patency of hemodynamic measurements obtained intraoperatively with a pulsed Doppler flowmeter in arterial and venous coronary bypass grafts was assessed.

The mean flow measured intraoperatively in 168 intact grafts was 60 ± 3 mL/min (range 9 to 230 mL/min), and the resistance was 1.8 ± 0.1 PRU (range 0.3 to 9.0 PRU). The mean flow was 36 ± 5 mL/min (range 2 to 107 mL/min), and the resistance was 5.9 ± 2.0 PRU (range 0.6 to 46.0 PRU) in 25 grafts found occluded at angiographic evaluation. Thus, abnormal hemodynamic values of arterial and venous bypass grafts detected intraoperatively are associated with later graft occlusion. Furthermore, multivariate analysis performed on graft-related hemodynamic variables selected increased resistance as the only independent variable that correlated with postoperative occlusion. Velocity curve patterns had a low specificity for postoperative graft patency and were more discriminating for grafts implanted into the left coronary system. In contrast, the predictive value for late stenosis could not be demonstrated for any of the graft-specific parameters.

Multivariate analysis (generalized estimating equations), including analysis of graft hemodynamic variables, the nature of the bypass conduit, and coronary- and patient-related variables, was carried out. Three independent variables were associated with a reduced patency rate: preoperative cardiogenic shock (P=0.040); increasing interval of control angiography (P=0.006); and increased resistance as measured in the graft (P=0.012).

In conclusion, the prognosis for mid-term patency of aortocoronary bypass grafts depends largely on the intraoperative hemodynamic status. Pulsed Doppler flowmeter measurements can designate grafts at risk of failure that will require close follow-up.

References

1. Walker JA, Friedberg DH, Flemma RG, et al. Determinants of angiographic patency of aortocoronary vein bypass grafts. Circulation 1972; 45,46:(suppl I):86–95.
2. Grondin CM, Meere C, Castonguay YR. Blood flow through aorta-to-coronary artery bypass grafts and early postoperative patency. Ann Thorac Surg 1971; 12:574–583.
3. Moran JM, Chen PY, Reinlander HF. Coronary hemodynamics following aorta-coronary bypass grafts. Arch Surg 1971; 103:539–549.
4. Björk VO, Ekeström S, Henze A, Ivert T, Landou C. Early and late patency of aortocoronary vein grafts. Scand J Thorac Cardiovasc Surg 1981; 15:11–21.
5. Balderman SC, Moran JM, Scanlon PJ, Pifarré R. Predictors of late aorta-coronary graft patency: intraoperative phasic flow versus angiography. J Thorac Cardiovasc Surg 1980; 79:724–728.
6. De Rijbel RJ, Schipperheyn JJ. The use of electromagnetic flow measurements for detection of early stenosis in aortocoronary bypass grafts. Ann Thorac Surg 1981; 31:402–408.
7. Simpson IA, Spyt TJ, Wheatley DJ, Cobbe SM. Assessment of coronary artery bypass graft flow by intraoperative Doppler ultrasound technique. Cardiovasc Res 1988; 22:484–488.
8. Bandyk DF, Galbraith TA, Haasler GB, Almassi GH. Blood flow velocity of internal mammary artery and saphenous vein grafts to the coronary arteries. J Surg Res 1988; 44:342–351.
9. Louagie YAG, Haxhe JP, Jamart J, Buche M, Schoevaerdts JC. Intraoperative assessment of coronary artery bypass grafts using a pulsed Doppler flowmeter. Ann Thorac Surg 1994; 58:742–749.
10. Louagie Y, Jamart J, Buche M, Eucher P, Van San P, et al. Intraoperative hemodynamic assessment of gastroepiploic artery and saphenous vein bypass grafts: a comparative study. J Thorac Cardiovasc Surg 1999; 118:330–338.
11. Louagie Y, Buche M, Eucher P, Schoevaerdts J-C. Intraoperative flow measurements in gastroepiploic grafts using pulsed Doppler. Eur J Cardiothorac Surg 1999; 15:240–246.
12. Louagie Y, Brockmann C, Jamart J, Schroeder E, Buche M, et al. Pulsed Doppler intraoperative flow assessment and midterm coronary graft patency. Ann Thorac Surg 1998; 66:1282–1288.
13. Liang KY, Zeger SL. Longitudinal data analysis using generalized linear models. Biometrika 1986; 73:13–22.
14. Davis CS. A computer program for regression analysis of repeated measures using generalized estimating equations. Comput Methods Programs Biomed 1993; 40:15–31.
15. Metz CE. ROC methodology in radiologic imaging. Invest Radiol 1986; 21:720–733.

16. Louagie YAG, Haxhe JP, Buche M, Schoevaerdts J-C. Intraoperative electro-magnetic flowmeter measurements in coronary artery bypass grafts. Ann Thorac Surg 1994; 57:357–364.
17. Frey RR, Bruschke AVG, Vermeulen FE. Serial angiographic evaluation 1 year and 9 years after aorta-coronary bypass: a study of 55 patients chosen at random. J Thorac Cardiovasc Surg 1984; 87:167–174.
18. Lytle BW, Loop FD, Cosgrove DM, Ratliff NB, Easley K, et al. Long-term (5 to 12 years) serial studies of internal mammary artery and saphenous vein coronary bypass grafts. J Thorac Cardiovasc Surg 1985; 89:248–258.
19. Zeff RH, Kongtahworn C, Iannone LA, Gordon DF, Brown TM, et al. Internal mammary artery versus saphenous vein graft to the left anterior descending coronary artery: prospective randomized study with 10-year follow-up. Ann Thorac Surg 1988; 45:533–536.
20. van der Meer J, Hillege HL, van Gilst WH, Brutel de la Rivière A, Dunselman PHJM, et al. for the CABADAS Research Group. A comparison of internal mammary artery and saphenous vein grafts after coronary artery bypass surgery: no differences in 1-year occlusion rates and clinical outcome. Circulation 1994; 90:2367–2374.
21. Crosby IK, Wellons HA Jr, Taylor GJ, Maffeo CJ, Beller GA, et al. Critical analysis of the preoperative and operative predictors of aortocoronary bypass patency. Ann Surg 1981; 193:743–751.
22. Manninen HI, Jaakkola P, Suhonen M, Rehnberg S, Vuorenniemi R, et al. Angiographic predictors of graft patency and disease progression after coronary artery bypass grafting with arterial and venous grafts. Ann Thorac Surg 1998; 66:1289–1294.
23. Gurné O, Buche M, Chenu P, Paquay JL, Pelgrim JP, et al. Quantitative angiographic follow-up study of the free inferior epigastric coronary bypass graft. Circulation 1994; 90:148–154.
24. Nakao T, Kawaue Y. Effect of coronary revascularization with the right gastroepiploic artery: comparative examination of angiographic findings in the early postoperative period. J Thorac Cardiovasc Surg 1993; 106:149–153.
25. Hashimoto H, Isshiki T, Ikari Y, Hara K, Saeki F, et al. Effects of competitive blood flow on arterial graft patency and diameter: medium-term postoperative follow-up. J Thorac Cardiovasc Surg 1996; 111:399–407.
26. Koiwa Y, Bahn RC, Ritman EL. Regional myocardial volume perfused by the coronary artery branch: estimation in vivo. Circulation 1986; 74:157–163.
27. Jaber SF, Koenig SC, BhaskerRao B, VanHimbergen DJ, Spence PA. Can visual assessment of flow waveform morphology detect anastomotic error in off-pump coronary artery bypass grafting? Eur J Cardiothorac Surg 1998; 14:476–479.
28. Jaber SF, Koenig SC, Bhasker Rao B, VanHimbergen DJ, Cerrito P, et al. Role of graft flow measurement technique in anastomotic quality assessment in minimally invasive CABG. Ann Thorac Surg 1998; 66:1087–1092.
29. Koenig SC, VanHimbergen DJ, Jaber SF, Ewert DL, Cerrito P, et al. Spectral analysis of graft flow for anastomotic error detection in off-pump CABG. Eur J Cardiothorac Surg 1999; 16(suppl 1):S83–S87.
30. D'Ancona G, Karamanoukian HL, Salerno TA, Schmid S, Bergsland J. Graft revision after transit time flow measurement (TTFM) in off-pump coronary artery bypass grafting (CABG). Eur J Cardiothorac Surg 1999; 452 (abstract).
31. Lytle BW, Loop FD, Taylor PC, Simpfendorfer C, Kramer JR, et al. Vein graft disease: the clinical impact of stenoses in saphenous vein bypass grafts to coronary arteries. J Thorac Cardiovasc Surg 1992; 103:831–840.

11

Transit Time Flow Measurements:

From Bench To Bedside

Beat H. Walpoth, MD, Guido Beldi, MD,
Andreas Bosshard, MD, Otto M. Hess, MD,
Thierry Carrel, MD

Introduction

Evaluation of coronary artery bypass grafts by intraoperative flow measurements has become a new standard in cardiovascular surgery. The possibility to intraoperatively detect and correct technical imperfections of coronary bypass grafts has gained considerable interest.[1–4] The transit time flow method is a simple and cost-effective technology that helps to reduce postoperative ischemia and infarction, and hence, morbidity and mortality.[3–5] In the era of total arterial revascularization and off-pump surgery, the control of the anastomoses is of utmost importance since arterial conduits are smaller and sensitive to vasospasm.[6,7] Recently the transit time method has been introduced into cardiovascular surgery for assessing coronary bypass flow.[8–10] The technique has been validated in several experimental and clinical studies.[8,9,11,12] The practical value of this method has been shown in quality assessments of bypass grafts during cardiovascular surgery.[2,4]

Validation of the Technique

Three different transit time flow systems have been tested in our laboratory under in vitro conditions using an artificial flow model.[13] Venous

From: D'Ancona G, Karamanoukian HL, Ricci M, Salerno TA, Bergsland J (eds). *Intraoperative Graft Patency Verification in Cardiac and Vascular Surgery.* © Futura Publishing Company, Armonk, NY, 2001.

and arterial segments were perfused with either physiological saline or blood (hematocrit 25% and 40%), respectively, at body or room temperature, using a roller pump with pulsatile flow (flow rates between 0 and 350 mL/min). The following 3 systems were evaluated:

1. CardioMed from Medi-Stim, Oslo, Norway (Model CM 400S)
2. Transonic Inc., Ithaca, USA (Model T 206)
3. Triton Technologies, San Diego, USA (Model 257 system 6).

All 3 systems showed an excellent correlation (r=0.93 for CardioMed, r=0.95 for Transonic, and r=0.93 for Triton), with true flow (blood sampling) after second order correction (i.e., mathematical correction using the regression equation obtained from the uncorrected transit time flow and true flow). This correction allowed adjusting for the under- or overestimations of the true flow by the transit time technique. System 1 (MediStim) and 2 (Transonic) showed only minor deviation from true value after second order correction. System 3 (Triton) showed, during online registration (Fig. 1, left-hand panel), a significant overestimation of the arterial flow and a significant underestimation of the venous flow. Thus, for system 3, the unsatisfactory correlation (r=0.71) was improved to a good correlation (r=0.93) after second order correction. Temperature, hematocrit, and use of saline or blood had no significant influence on transit time flow measurements. These results compare well with published data in vitro, and experimental or clinical results.[13] From this study, we concluded that systems 1 and 2 showed excellent correlation to true flow, whereas system 3 demonstrated significant deviations from true flow values. Proper validation with mathematical corrections also yielded a reliable measurement for system 3. Due to its easy and fast applicability and excellent reproducibility, transit time flow measurement appears to be the method of choice for intraoperative flow measurement. This may be important for quality control and outcome studies.

Detection of Flow Differences Between Venous and Arterial Bypass Grafts

Clinical application of the transit time technique includes flow measurements of venous (SVG) and arterial (IMA) bypass grafts after completion of coronary anastomosis and following weaning from cardiopulmonary bypass. Graft flow measurements were obtained in the proximal third of the graft using 4–5 mm probes for venous and 3–4 mm probes for arterial grafts (CardioMed, Medi-Stim, AS, Oslo, Norway). Flow measurements were performed at rest (baseline) and after maximal vasodilation

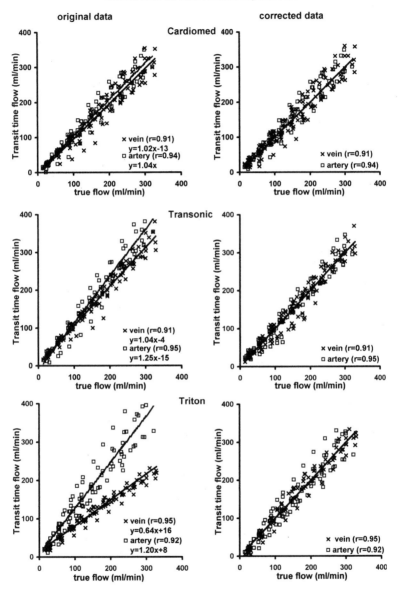

Figure 1. Comparison of 3 commercially available flow meters (CardioMed, Transonic, Triton) using blood sampling as reference technique. Flow data were obtained between 0 and 350 mL for arterial (□) and venous (X) bypass grafts: regression analysis of the 3 flow systems showing excellent correlation after second order correction. (Reproduced with permission of the Annals of Thoracic Surgery.[1])

with adenosine (25 µg/kg/min) injected directly into the left ventricle (Fig. 2). Resting and maximal flow as well as coronary flow reserve (CFR: maximal flow/resting flow) were measured in all patients.

Mean flow at rest (n=25) was significantly higher in SVG (63 ± 29 mL/min) than in IMA grafts (32 ± 11 mL/min; P< 0.001) (Fig. 3). However, CFR was similar in both bypass grafts (1.7 ± 0.5 for SVG and 1.4 ± 0.5 for IMA), but significantly lower than in normal controls (CFR ≥2.5).[14,15]

Despite a larger perfusion territory (angiographic determination: IMA 97 ± 53 g versus SVG 70 ± 70 g; ns), coronary bypass flow was significantly lower in the IMA grafts when compared to the SV grafts.[16] This mismatch between perfusion territory and bypass flow can be explained by several mechanisms (technical failures, vasospasm, competitive flow through the native artery, myocardial stunning) but may also be due to initial adaptation of the IMA to the flow requirements of the revascularized myocardium. Preliminary data have shown that 12 months after revascularization flow has doubled and flow reserve has returned to normal in the IMA grafts, suggesting that the arterial grafts have adapted to the flow requirements of the myocardium (positive vascular remodeling).[17] The exact mechanisms of this adaptation are not known but are thought to be due to flow or NO-mediated factors.

Detection of Early Graft Failure During Myocardial Revascularization

Low coronary bypass flow due to technical failure is of major concern in coronary artery bypass surgery and may be associated with myocardial infarction and pump failure.[14,15] Thus, early recognition of low bypass flow is essential to prevent these complications and should alert the surgeon to look for technical imperfections in the bypass. In the past, the proper functioning of a bypass graft was assessed on the basis of hemodynamics, ECG tracings, and evaluation of ventricular contractility. Malfunctioning grafts were suspected when difficulty in weaning the patient from cardiopulmonary bypass was encountered.[15,17] Techniques other than flow measurements for detection of bypass failure include transesophageal echocardiography or intraoperative angiography.[18,19] However, intraoperative bypass flow measurements using transit time flow methods are simple, easy to perform, and give reliable (physiological) information on myocardial perfusion. In a series of 46 high-risk patients with hemodynamic instability, severely reduced left ventricular function, and/or diffuse coronary artery disease, transit time flow measurements were performed[1] for intraoperative graft patency verification (Fig. 4). In 3

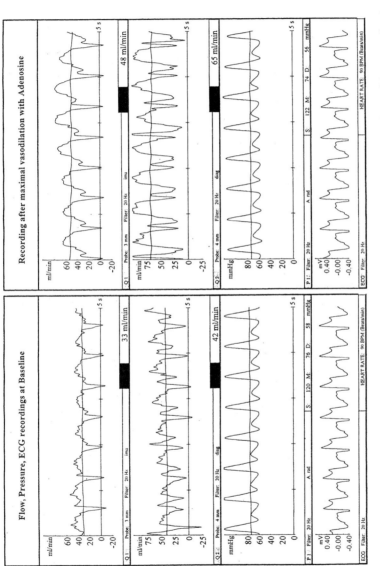

Figure 2. Original registration of a venous and an arterial bypass graft before and after maximal vasodilation with adenosine. Resting flow was 33 (IMA) and 42 (SVG) mL/min, hyperemic flow 48 (IMA) and 65 (SVG) mL/min. Coronary flow reserve was 1.5 for both the IMA and SVG in this patient.

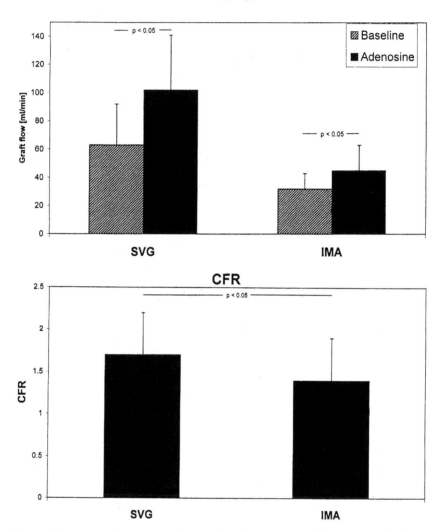

Figure 3. Intraoperative coronary bypass flow in 25 patients after weaning from cardiopulmonary bypass (top). Data are shown at baseline and after maximal vasodilation with adenosine for venous (left) and arterial (right) grafts. CFR of venous and arterial bypass grafts (bottom). There was no difference in CFR although bypass flow in SVG doubled flow in IMA grafts. Mean value ±1 SD; *P< 0.05.

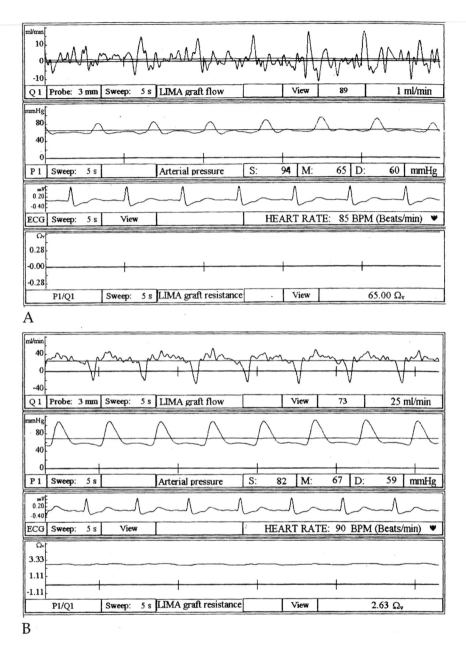

Figure 4. Transit time flow measurement of the left IMA bypass to the LAD coronary artery. Shown are: coronary bypass flow (Q1; top signal), aortic pressure (P1; second signal), electrocardiogram (ECG; third signal), vascular resistance (P1/Q1; fourth signal). The top panel shows data during bypass failure (dissection) and the bottom panel shows data after revision of the distal anastomosis. Flow increased from 1 mL/min to 25 mL/min. (Reproduced with permission of the Annals of Thoracic Surgery.[1])

patients, a low-flow situation (0.5 ± 0.7 mL/min) with a high coronary resistance and pulsatility index was found in one of the arterial bypass grafts. The reason for the low-flow situation was an IMA dissection in one patient, an obstructing IMA intimal flap in another, and an intramural hematoma with compression of the vessel lumen in the third patient.

In all 3 patients the distal anastomosis was revised while the patient was back on cardiopulmonary bypass. After revision, flow increased to 16 ± 10 mL/min (P<0.02). Pulsatility index, diastolic backflow, and vascular resistance reached values comparable to those in the control group (Table 1).

IMA flow values in these 3 patients were, however, lower than those of the IMA grafts in the control patients (Table 1). This was probably due to vasospasm after reclamping the aorta or was the result of excessive operative manipulation of the IMA. Another reason may be the lower mean arterial pressure after revision as compared to the control patients. Low bypass flow due to early graft failure is associated with a high risk of myocardial infarction. Intraoperative detection of graft failure remains important to ensure early and long-term patency of the conduits. In a high-risk group, 7% (3 of 46) of all patients showed an early graft failure, i.e., 3 out of 129 grafts (2% of all grafts). Early intraoperative recognition of bypass failure allowed the surgeon to revise the anastomoses immediately, while the sternum was still open.[1-4,20] Similar data on transit time flow measurements have been reported by other groups, with intraoperative revisions close to 8%. Postoperative outcome was, however, excellent in these patients.[4]

Table 1
Flow and Pressure Data of IMA Grafts in Three Patients with Graft Failure Before and After Operative Revision

Variables	Occlusion	Revision	Controls
Bypass flow (mL/min)	0.5 ± 0.7	16 ± 10 *	33 ± 27 **
Mean arterial pressure (mm Hg)	69 ± 7	68 ± 2	80 ± 9 **
Vascular resistance (mm Hg/mL/min)	138 ± 10	5 ± 2 *	4 ± 3
Pulsatility index	147 ± 96	3 ± 2 *	3 ± 2
Diastolic backflow (% insufficiency)	68 ± 35	8 ± 9 *	6 ± 7
Systolic/diastolic flow ratio (%)	—	61 ± 6	47 ± 15
Systolic/diastolic time ratio	62 ± 7	59 ± 16	57 ± 10
Diastolic filling pattern	no	yes	yes

Control data are from 43 patients with coronary artery disease.
The various indices are explained in the text (*P< 0.05 to failure; **P< 0.05 to revision).

Our experience with transit time flow measurements has been very fruitful and we would make the following recommendations:

1. Bypass flow measurements should be done in all patients undergoing arterial bypass grafting and especially in those estimated to be at increased risk because of small vessels, poor runoff, and off-pump coronary surgery.
2. Assessment should be done at rest and after maximal vasodilatation in patients with low-flow situations and in all cases with suspected vasospasm. Bypass grafts with low baseline flows (<10 mL/min) or no flow improvement during vasodilation should be reevaluated intraoperatively.
3. Early recognition of graft failure is cost-effective and may prevent hemodynamic instability and perioperative myocardial infarction, reducing length of stay in the intensive care unit and improving the patient's outcome.

References

1. Walpoth BH, Bosshard A, Genyk I, Kipfer B, Berdat PA, et al. Transit-time flow measurement for detection of early graft failure during myocardial revascularization. Ann Thorac Surg 1998; 63:12–17.
2. Walpoth BH, Bosshard A, Kipfer B, Berdat PA, Althaus U, et al. Failed coronary artery bypass anastomosis detected by intraoperative coronary flow measurement. Eur J Cardiothorac Surg 1998; 14:76–81.
3. Carrel T, Kujawski T, Zünd G, et al. The internal mammary artery malperfusion syndrome: incidence, treatment and angiographic verification. Eur J Cardiothorac Surg 1995; 9:190–197.
4. D'Ancona G, Karamanoukian HL, Ricci M, Schmid S, Bergsland J, et al. Graft revision after transit time flow measurement in off-pump coronary artery bypass grafting. Eur J Cardiothorac Surg 2000; 17:287–293.
5. Alderman EL. Angiographic correlates of graft patency and relationship to clinical outcomes. Ann Thorac Surg 1996; 62:22–25.
6. Calafiore AM, Di Giammarco G, Teodori G, et al. Left anterior descending coronary artery grafting via left anterior small thoracotomy without cardiopulmonary bypass. Ann Thorac Surg 1996; 61:1658–1667.
7. Caputo M, Nicolini F, Franciosi G, Galloti R. Coronary artery spasm after coronary artery bypass grafting. Eur J Cardiothorac Surg 1999; 15:545–548.
8. Walpoth BH, Mohadjer A, Gersbach P, Rogulenko R, Walpoth BN, et al. Intraoperative internal mammary artery transit-time flow measurements: comparative evaluation of two surgical pedicle preparation techniques. Eur J Cardiothorac Surg 1996; 10:1064–1070.
9. Canver CHC, Dame NA. Ultrasonic assessment of internal thoracic artery graft flow in the revascularized heart. Ann Thorac Surg 1990; 58:135–138.
10. Louagie YAG, Haxhe JP, Jamart J, Gurne O, Buche M, et al. Perioperative hemodynamic study of left internal mammary artery grafts. Thorac Cardiovasc Surg 1995; 43:27–34.

11. Laustsen J, Pedersen EM, Terp K, Steinbrüchel D, Kure HH, et al. Validation of a new transit time ultrasound flowmeter in man. Eur J Vasc Endovasc Surg 1996; 12:91–96.
12. Barnea O, Santamore WP. Intraoperative monitoring of IMA flow: what does it mean? Ann Thorac Surg 1997; 63:12–17.
13. Beldi G, Bosshard A, Hess OM, Althaus U, Walpoth BH. Transit time flow measurement: experimental validation and comparison of three different systems. Ann Thorac Surg 2000; 70:212–217.
14. Barner HB. Coronary flow reserve: physiologically important, operatively altered, and clinically emerging. Ann Thorac Surg 1988; 45:469–470.
15. von Segesser L. Inadequate flow after internal mammary artery-coronary artery revascularization. Thorac Cardiovasc Surg 1987; 35:352–354.
16. Mandinov L, Kaufmann P, Maier W, Hess OM. Flow-dependent vasodilation in the coronary circulation: alterations in diseased states. Semin Interven Cardiol 1998; 3:5–12.
17. Flemma RJ, Singh TM, Tector AJ, Lepley D, Frazier BL. Comparative hemodynamic properties of vein and mammary artery in coronary bypass operations. Ann Thorac Surg 1975; 20:619–627.
18. Caretta Q, Voci P, Bilotta F, Mercanti C, Marino B. Intraoperative detection of coronary artery graft occlusion by myocardial contrast echocardiography. J Cardiothorac Vasc Anesth 1994; 8:206–208.
19. Spence PA, Lust RM, Zeri RS, Jolly SR, Metha PM, et al. Competitive flow from a fully patent coronary artery does not limit acute mammary graft flow. Ann Thorac Surg 1992; 54:21–25.
20. Bosshard A, Carrel T, Kipfer B, Berdat P, Neidhart C, et al. Flow mismatch of arterial and venous coronary bypass graft. Submitted for publication.

Appendix

Exercise in Graft Patency Verification in Coronary Artery Surgery

Susan Schmid, RN, Giuseppe D'Ancona, MD,
Hratch Karamanoukian, MD, Marco Ricci, MD,
Tomas A. Salerno, MD, Jacob Bergsland, MD

Introduction

The theoretical basis of "flowmetry" has already been presented extensively in previous chapters of this book. Intraoperative graft patency verification has a strong scientific background supported by in vitro and in vivo experiments. In daily clinical practice, surgeons have to deal with situations that require immediate solutions. Practical rules, derived from the empirical observation of different cases, should be applied to expedite the decision-making process and to assure good outcome of the surgical procedure. In this appendix, we will try to give some guidelines to correctly interpret the transit time flow measurement (TTFM) findings. This is mainly a "practical exercise session" and, for this reason, is separated from the rest of the book chapters. Fourteen clinical cases are reported in a standard format, focusing on the different intraoperative TTFM findings. Differences between functional and nonfunctional grafts are presented. The suggestions and guidelines given in this appendix are derived from 4 years of clinical work on more than 900 patients. We hope our "learning experience" will help the readers avoid fatal mistakes in their daily practice. Although a lot could be taught about flow measurement, most of the confidence with the TTFM technology should be progressively acquired in the operating room. The flowmeter is not a "magic bullet" that can be sporadically used to solve the most complicated clinical situations. On the contrary, intraoperative graft patency verification should be performed routinely to fully understand its potential and to improve perioperative results of both off-pump and on-pump coronary surgery.

—Giuseppe D'Ancona, MD

From: D'Ancona G, Karamanoukian HL, Ricci M, Salerno TA, Bergsland J (eds). *Intraoperative Graft Patency Verification in Cardiac and Vascular Surgery.* © Futura Publishing Company, Armonk, NY, 2001.

Case #1

Clinical History

AF is a 77-year-old white male with no history of myocardial infarction (MI), rheumatic heart disease, congestive heart failure (CHF), or angina. Comorbidities included:

♦ Severe chronic obstructive pulmonary disease (COPD)
♦ Hypertension (HTN)
♦ Noninsulin-dependent diabetes mellitus (NIDDM)

Ventriculography

Left ventricular ejection fraction (LVEF) was 50%, with mild mitral regurgitation.

Angiographic Findings

The left anterior descending (LAD) coronary artery showed a proximal 85–90% stenosis with dense calcifications just after the origin of a mildly narrowed (35%) major diagonal (D) branch. The left circumflex (LCX) coronary artery was occluded with the major obtuse marginal (OM) artery filling by collaterals. The proximal right coronary artery (RCA) showed a fractured plaque with an 80–85% stenosis.

Operation

The patient underwent off-pump coronary artery bypass grafting (OPCABG) via median sternotomy. Bypasses were performed as follows:

♦ Left internal mammary artery (LIMA) → LAD
♦ Saphenous vein graft (SVG) → RCA

The LAD had a 1.5-mm lumen. The LIMA was anastomosed to the LAD just before the origin of the D2 branch. A 7.0 Prolene running suture was used for the anastomosis.

Transit Time Flowmeter (TTFM) Findings:

PI:	2.2	Insufficiency:	2.7%
		Mean flow without proximal snare:	33.1 mL/min

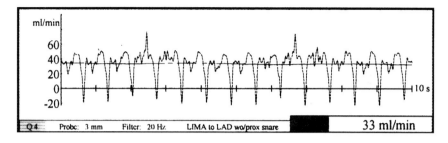

Figure 1. LIMA → LAD without snare, mean flow 33.1 mL/min.

TTFM (continued)

PI: 2.2   Insufficiency: 1.7%
              Mean flow with
                  proximal snare: 39.7 mL/min

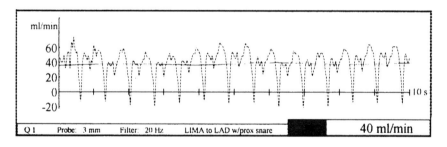

Figure 2. LIMA → LAD with snare, mean flow 39.7 mL/min.

TTFM showed a very good diastolic flow pattern with a low pulsatility index (PI) value and minimal insufficiency. Measurements with and without proximal snare were both adequate. Probe-graft contact was adequate as shown by the indicator in the right lower corner of Figure 2. Mean flow value was within average (35 mL/min ± 15 mL).

TTFM of the SVG → RCA graft was also adequate. The LIMA → LAD was remeasured prior to chest closure before protamine was given. The following were the findings:

PI: 12.7   Insufficiency: 21.0%
              Mean flow without
                  proximal snare: 2.2 mL/min

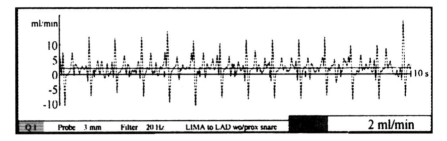

Figure 3. LIMA → LAD without snare, mean flow 2.2 mL/min.

Comment

This second measurement showed a very low (2 mL/min), mainly systolic flow in the LIMA. The PI was significantly elevated (>5). On the basis of these findings, it was decided to revise the anastomosis.

Findings at Revision

A flap with a small dissection and thrombus was found at the distal end of the LIMA. The distal end of the LIMA was excised and reanastomosed to the LAD with these final findings:

PI: 1.2   Insufficiency: 0.0%
              Mean flow with
                  proximal snare   29.3 mL/min

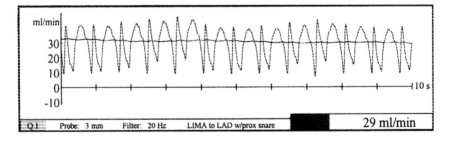

Figure 4. LIMA → LAD with snare, mean flow 29.3 mL/min.

PI: 2.6   Insufficiency: 4.3%
              Mean flow without
                  proximal snare   15.0 mL/min

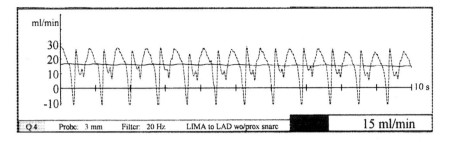

Figure 5. LIMA→ LAD without snare, mean flow 15.0 mL/min.

Comment

TTFM findings seem to have returned to normal. A typical LIMA → LAD flow pattern with a mainly diastolic curve is shown in Figure 5. PI is low (<5). Insufficiency is low and mean flow is within average (35 mL/min ± 15). A significant competitive flow from the native LAD can be deducted by the decrease in actual flow through the LIMA when the coronary snare is released (from 29 mL/min with snare to 15 mL/min without snare).

Patient Outcome

AF's LIMA → LAD graft had to be revised due to a flap, and small dissection of the distal LIMA. He was discharged 5 days after surgery with no elevation in CPK(MB) values. At 3-month follow-up, the patient has begun cardiac rehabilitation without complaints of chest pain or shortness of breath (SOB).

Case #2

Clinical History

SC is 45-year-old white male with a medical history positive for recent onset of MI.

Ventriculography

An apical akinesis with preserved left ventricular systolic function (EF 60%) was noted.

Angiographic Findings

The LAD had an 80–90% stenosis just after the origin of the D2 branch. The distal LAD had a 50% stenosis. The OM1 had a 90% stenosis at its origin. The proximal and mid-portion of the RCA had moderate diffuse irregularities that accounted for a 60% stenosis. The distal RCA had a 60–70% stenosis just prior to the origin of the posterior descending coronary artery (PDA).

Operation

The patient underwent OPCABG via median sternotomy. Bypasses were performed as follows:

- LIMA → LAD
- SVG → RCA (proximal RCA)
- SVG → OM1
- SVG → RCA (distal RCA)

The SVG was anastomosed to the distal portion of the RCA, which had a 2.0-mm lumen. A 7.0 Prolene running suture was used.

TTFM Findings

Upon completion of LIMA → LAD, SVG → OM1, TTFM revealed no problems with the grafts. The first measurement of the SVG → RCA had the following pattern:

PI: 29.7   Insufficiency: 58%
                 Mean flow without
                     proximal snare: 5.9 mL/min

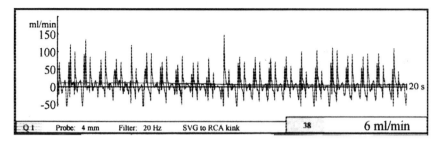

Figure 6. SVG → RCA without snare, mean flow 5.9 mL/min.

TTFM showed a continuous systolic spike, with an elevated PI (29.7) and a low mean flow (6 mL/min).

Findings at Revision

At surgical revision, the distal end of the SVG was found to be twisted. The anastomosis was disconnected and reconstructed carefully. Flow was remeasured. These findings were reported:

PI: 1.0   Insufficiency: 0.0%
            Mean flow without
                proximal snare: 51.6 mL/min

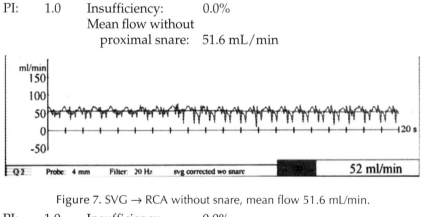

Figure 7. SVG → RCA without snare, mean flow 51.6 mL/min.

PI: 1.0   Insufficiency: 0.0%
            Mean flow with
                proximal snare: 56.2 mL/min

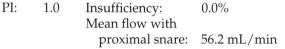
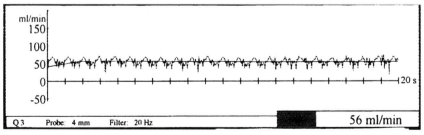

Figure 8. SVG → RCA with snare, mean flow 56.2 mL/min.

Comment

After surgical revision, both flow patterns with and without snare showed a continuous diastolic curve with low PIs (1.0 and 1.0). Mean flow values were acceptable at 51.6 mL/min and 56.2 mL/min.

Before chest closure TTFM was again used to check the revised graft (SVG → RCA). These findings were reported:

PI: 13.4   Insufficiency: 25.0%
               Mean flow with
                  proximal snare: 11.2 mL/min

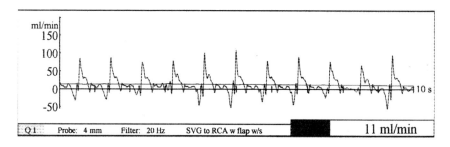

Figure 9. SVG → RCA with snare, mean flow 11.2 mL/min.

PI: 66.4   Insufficiency: 78.7%
               Mean flow without
                  proximal snare   1.9 mL/min

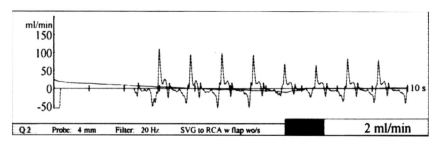

Figure 10. SVG → RCA without snare, mean flow 1.9 mL/min.

TTFM showed a sharp systolic spike with very little diastolic curve with and without proximal snare. PIs were above normal limits (13.4 and 66.4). Mean flows were unacceptable (11 mL/min and 2 mL/min) if compared to the 2 previous measurements.

The anastomosis was revised for the second time.

Findings at Revision

An intimal flap was noticed in the native vessel after having performed a longer arteriotomy. A new anastomosis was constructed.
New TTFM findings were reported:

PI: 2.4   Insufficiency: 3.1%
                  Mean flow with
                      proximal snare: 23.4 mL/min

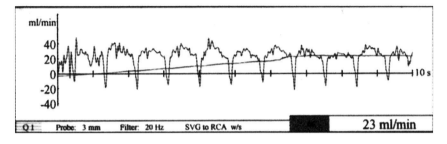

Figure 11. SVG → RCA with snare, mean flow 23.4 mL/min.

PI: 2.3   Insufficiency: 3.2%
                  Mean flow without
                      proximal snare: 26.3 mL/min

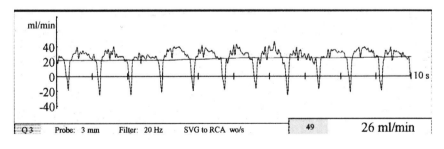

Figure 12. SVG → RCA without snare, mean flow 26.3 mL/min.

TTFM showed the typical round diastolic flow curve, without systolic spikes. PIs were well within normal limits (2.4 and 2.3). Mean flow with and without snare was not as high as the previous one (51 and 56 mL/min) but was more than adequate.

Patient Outcome

SC's SVG → RCA graft had to be revised twice. The first time a graft "twist" was found, and the second time an intimal flap in the native coronary was discovered. Postoperatively there was no elevation in CPK(MB). SC was discharged without complications. He underwent a postoperative stress test at 1 month, demonstrating no signs of myocardial ischemia. He continues to do well 3 years after surgery.

Case #3

Clinical History

BV is a 59-year-old white male who denied any history of angina or myocardial infarction. No previous surgical history was reported. Symptoms included diffuse diaphoresis and SOB. Family history was positive for coronary artery disease (CAD).

Ventriculography

The left ventricular EF% was within normal limits.

Angiographic Findings

The left main was 90–95% stenosed. OM1 showed a 60% stenosis. The RCA had a proximal 40% plaque with a normal posterior descending coronary artery.

Operation

The patient underwent OPCABG via median sternotomy. Use of cardiopulmonary bypass (CPB) was necessary to revise the OM1 graft. The following bypasses were performed:

- LIMA → LAD
- SVG → DIAG
- SVG → RCA
- SVG → OM1

The OM1 had a lumen of 1.5 mm. The SV was anastomosed using a 7.0 Prolene running suture.

TTFM Findings

PI: 22.9   Insufficiency: 56.2%
                   Mean flow without
                       proximal snare: 7.0 mL/min

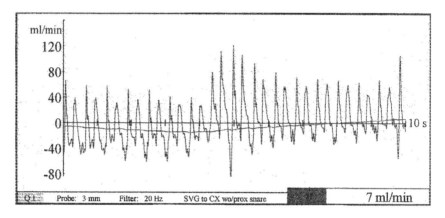

Figure 13. SVG → CX without snare, mean flow 7.0 mL/min.

Comment

The curve showed a mainly systolic flow pattern with high spikes and PI values. A second measurement was performed to exclude spasm or air in the graft. Findings remained unchanged:

PI: 12.5   Insufficiency: 44.5%
                Mean flow without
                    proximal snare: 13.0 mL/min

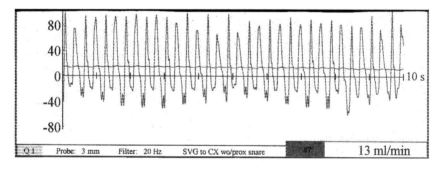

Figure 14. SVG → CX without snare, mean flow 13.0 mL/min.

Elevated PIs, continuous systolic flow pattern, low mean flow, and high insufficiency convinced the surgeon to redo the graft. CPB was initiated due to hemodynamic instability while re-exposing the OM1 coronary artery.

Findings at Revision

A stitch compressing the toe of the graft was found to be the problem. After revision the following TTFM findings were recorded:

PI: 3.5   Insufficiency: 1.1
                Mean flow without
                    proximal snare: 19.6 mL/min

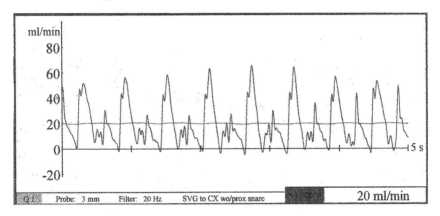

Figure 15. SVG → CX without snare, mean flow 19.6 mL/min.

Comment

The curve still had a large systolic spike, probably due to the high heart rate. On the contrary, a low PI (3.5) and a good component of diastolic flow (19.6 mL/min) were also noted, indicating a properly functioning graft. The graft was measured again before chest closure with the same results.

Patient Outcome

BV's SVG → CX graft had to be revised due to a compression stitch found at the toe of the anastomosis. Postoperatively there were no elevations in CPK(MB). BV was discharged without complications and in stable condition. His stress test at 1 month postoperative was normal.

Case #4

Clinical History

FJ is a 54-year-old white female with recent onset of chest tightness and SOB. Past surgical history was negative. Family history was positive for CAD.

Ventriculography

Left ventriculography demonstrated some hypokinesis of the inferior wall. Estimated overall EF% was 45%.

Angiographic Findings

The LM was normal. The LAD was significantly diseased just after the D2 branch with a 65–75% stenosis. D1 had a 40–50% narrowing. D2 was a moderately large vessel with a critical 90% narrowing. The CX was significantly diseased. The OM1 had a 20% proximal narrowing. The OM2 had a 99% narrowing with poor periphery.

Operation

The patient underwent OPCABG via median sternotomy. Bypasses were performed as follows:

- LIMA → LAD
- SVG→ DIAG
- SVG→ RCA

Upon completion of the LIMA → LAD and SVG → RCA, TTFM demonstrated no problems with these grafts. The CX was completely calcified and did not appear graftable. A SVG was anastomosed to D1. The vessel was found to have a 1.5-mm lumen and to be diffusely diseased. A 7.0 Prolene running suture was used to construct the anastomosis.

TTFM Findings

PI: 70.5   Insufficiency: 65.1%
                 Mean flow without
                    proximal snare: −0.6 mL/min

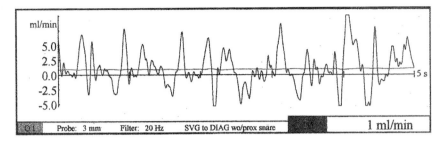

Figure 16. SVG → DIAG without snare, mean flow − 0.6 mL/min.

A second measurement was performed 5 minutes later to exclude any possible misreading due to air or spasm:

PI: 17.8   Insufficiency: 36.2%
              Mean flow without
                  proximal snare: 1.1 mL/min

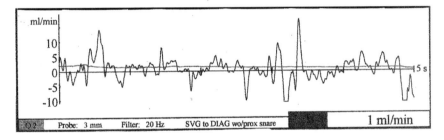

Figure 17. SVG → DIAG without snare, mean flow 1.1 mL/min.

Comment

Both TTFMs showed no diastolic flow pattern. Only systolic spikes were noted. PIs were elevated in both measurements (70.5 and 17.8). Insufficiency was elevated also. Mean flow was close to zero. Probes were without problems.

Findings at Revision

On the basis of TTFM findings, something was probably wrong with the D1 graft. The surgeon felt that the proximal anastomosis needed to be revised. After revision, TTFM findings were as follows:

PI: 11.8   Insufficiency: 23.1%
              Mean flow without
                  proximal snare: 3.0 mL/min

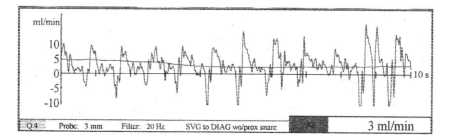

Figure 18. SVG → DIAG without snare, mean flow 3.0 mL/min.

TTFM (continued)

PI: 39.7   Insufficiency: 64%
                 Mean flow without
                    proximal snare: 0.9 mL/min

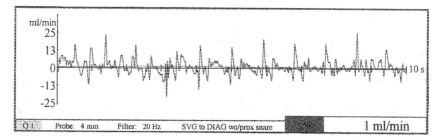

Figure 19. SVG → DIAG without snare, mean flow 0.9 mL/min.

Comment

There was a small amount of diastolic curve and no sharp systolic spikes in the second measurement; however, the flow was insignificant for a 1.5-mm diagonal. Also, the PIs were elevated in both measurements. Insufficiency was significant. Mean flow was low or nonexistent (3 mL/min and 1 mL/min). The distal anastomosis was then looked at as the source of the problem. At revision, the diagonal was found to be dissected. The distal anastomosis was reperformed, but TTFM findings remained unsatisfactory.

TTFM Findings

PI: 26.1   Insufficiency: 57%
                 Mean flow without
                    proximal snare: 1.3 mL/min

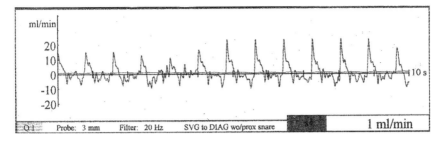

Figure 20. SVG → DIAG without snare, mean flow 1.3 mL/min.

Patient Outcome

FJ's SVG → DIAG had to be revised twice. After each anastomosis, there was still no flow in the bypass, and it was found that the DIAG had dissected. Postoperatively there was a slight elevation in CPK(MB), but overall the patient did well. She was discharged in stable condition. At 3-month follow-up, the patient did not have a stress test, but had no complaints of chest pain or SOB. She has resumed her normal activities.

Case #5

Clinical History

DR is a 48-year-old white male who was admitted for a non-Q wave MI. Comorbidities included:

- NIDDM
- Cigarette smoking history

Ventriculography

Left ventricular EF was 50%, with inferoapical akinesis.

Angiographic Findings

The LAD had a 70% lesion proximally and an 80% stenosis in its mid-zone, just before a first large D branch. In the mid- to distal LAD, there was a 40% plaque. The mid-portion of the RCA demonstrated an 80% stenosis. The OM1 had a 90% proximal stenosis. The CX had an 80% stenosis.

Operation

The patient underwent OPCABG via median sternotomy. Bypasses were performed as follows:

- LIMA → LAD
- RIMA → RCA
- SVG → OM1

TTFM demonstrated no problems with the LIMA → LAD and RIMA → RCA. SVG was anastomosed to a 2.5-mm OM1. A 7.0 Prolene running suture was used to construct the anastomosis.

TTFM Findings

PI: 69.0   Insufficiency: 82.7%
            Mean flow with
               proximal snare: 1.2 mL/min

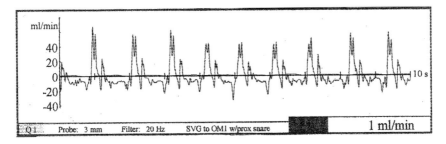

Figure 21. SVG → OM1 with snare, mean flow 1.2 mL/min.

Flow was remeasured after 10 minutes to exclude air or spasm:

PI: 65.2   Insufficiency: 83.7%
                   Mean flow with
                      proximal snare: 1.4 mL/min

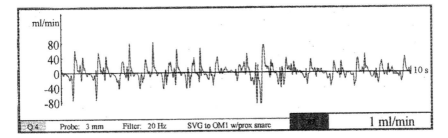

Figure 22. SVG → OM1 with snare, mean flow 1.4 mL/min.

PI: 48.1   Insufficiency: 75%
                   Mean flow without
                      proximal snare: 0.6 mL/min

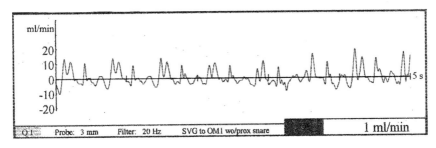

Figure 23. SVG → OM1 without snare, mean flow 0.6 mL/min.

Comment

TTFM showed sharp systolic spikes both with and without snare with no diastolic flow pattern. PIs were elevated in all measurements (69, 65.2, and 48.1). Insufficiency was elevated in every measurement, and mean flow was 1 mL/min or less. Probe function was normal.

Findings at Revision

Upon inspection, the graft was found to be too short. The anastomosis was redone more proximal on the OM1. TTFM results after the anastomosis was reperformed were as follows:

TTFM Findings (continued)

PI: 4.1   Insufficiency: 8.5%
              Mean flow without
                proximal snare: 62.0 mL/min

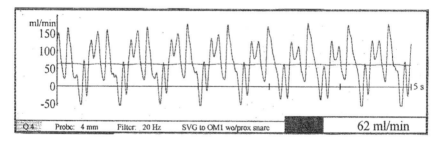

Figure 24. SVG → OM1 without snare, mean flow 62.0 mL/min.

Comment

TTFM showed a mainly diastolic curve pattern, without any systolic spikes. PI was within normal limits, and the insufficiency was considerably less. Mean flow was appropriate for a 2.5-mm vessel. The following TTFM measurement was taken before chest closure:

PI: 2.9   Insufficiency: 2.8%
              Mean flow without
                proximal snare: 65.8 mL/min

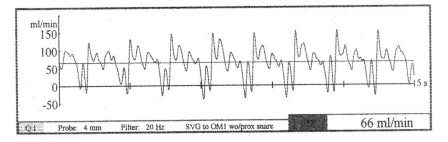

Figure 25. SVG → OM1 without snare, mean flow 65.8 mL/min.

TTFM showed an even better diastolic flow curve. Note that the curve has a step appearance in it. This is usually an indicator of air in the graft that can act like an obstruction. However, this graft improved only since the last measurement. The PI was lower (2.9), insufficiency came down even more, and the mean flow went up.

Patient Outcome

DR's SVG → OM1 graft, which was too short, had to be revised. The patient had no elevations of CPK(MB) postoperatively. He developed a postoperative mediastinitis treated with surgical debridement. Grafts were measured during sternal revision and were found to be patent. The patient was discharged in stable condition. At 3-month follow-up, he was without complaints. He denies chest pain or SOB. He is resuming his normal activities.

Case #6

Clinical History

SB is a 54-year-old white male who experienced chest discomfort during activity. Family history was positive for CAD.

Ventriculography

THe EF% was 50%, with mild inferobasal hypokinesia.

Angiographic Findings

The LAD had a 95% stenosis prior to and just after the D1 branch. The RCA was occluded after its origin, while the PDA visualized via collaterals from the left coronary artery. OM1 was occluded and filling via collaterals.

Operation

The patient underwent OPCABG via median sternotomy. Bypasses were performed as follows:

- LIMA → D1
- SVG → LAD
- SVG → RCA

The LIMA was grafted to the D1, which was a much larger vessel than the LAD. TTFM demonstrated no problems with the LIMA → D1, and the SVG → RCA. A segment of the SVG was anastomosed to a 1.5-mm LAD, using a 7.0 Prolene running suture.

TTFM Findings

PI: 1.8   Insufficiency: 0.0%
                Mean flow with
                    proximal snare: 11.4 mL/min

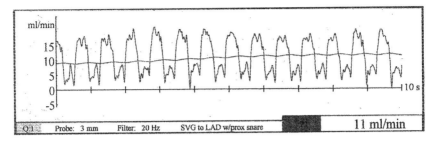

Figure 26. SVG → LAD with snare, mean flow 11.4 mL/min.

TTFM Findings (continued)

PI: 2.7 mL/min   Insufficiency: 1.4%
                     Mean flow without
                       proximal snare: 6.9 mL/min

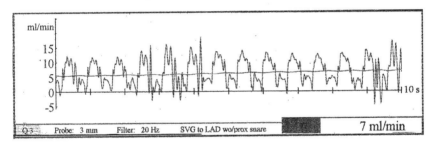

Figure 27. SVG → LAD without snare, mean flow 6.9 mL/min.

Comment

Both readings showed a very typical diastolic flow curve. Insufficiency was low or nonexsistent. PIs were well within normal limits. Mean flow with and without snare was relatively low. It was higher without the snare due to competition from the native vessel. However, this appeared to be a good TTFM curve. The surgeon was not happy with the mean flow and decided to redo the distal anastomosis.

Findings at Revision

The anastomosis was found to be free from technical imperfections. After a second anastomosis was constructed, the findings were as follows:

PI: 24   Insufficiency: 1.8%
             Mean flow with
               proximal snare: 13.7 mL/min

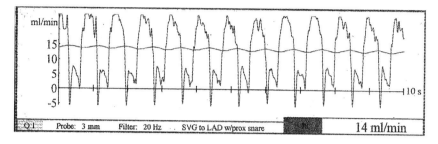

Figure 28. SVG → LAD with snare, mean flow 13.7 mL/min.

TTFM Findings (continued)

PI: 23   Insufficiency: 2.0%
              Mean flow without
                  proximal snare: 17.7 mL/min

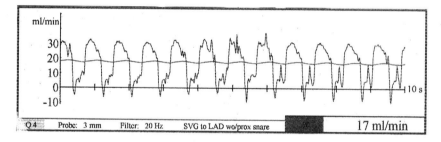

Figure 29. SVG → LAD without snare, mean flow 17.7 mL/min.

As before, both measurements had a nice diastolic flow curve, low insufficiency, and low PIs. Mean flow came up slightly but it may have come up even without redoing the graft. It is possible for a graft to demonstrate low mean flow despite being a perfectly functioning graft. Correct interpretation of TTFM findings should always take into consideration flow curve shape, PI value, and absolute flow value.

Patient Outcome

SB's graft (SVG → LAD) was revised due to low flow, despite normal flow curves and PI values. After revision, there was no significant change in flows. The patient had no elevation in CPKs postoperatively. He was discharged without complaints and in stable condition. At 3-month follow-up, the patient was symptom free.

Case #7

Clinical History

JB is a 66-year-old white male with unstable angina and CHF. Co-morbidities included:

- Previous CABG × 2
- Hepatitis C
- IDDM
- Chronic renal insufficiency

Ventriculography

Left ventriculogram showed inferior akinesis and anterior hypokine-sis with an EF of 20%.

Angiographic Findings

The arteriography showed a complete occlusion of the LAD and OM1. The RCA was completely occluded. A 90% stenosis of the old SVG to the LAD was also found.

Operation

The patient underwent a small left anterior thoracotomy for a single coronary artery bypass. The bypass was performed as follows:

- LIMA → SVG → LAD (H-graft)

The SVG was anastomosed laterally to the LIMA and then to a 2.0-mm LAD using a 7.0 Prolene running suture for the anastomosis.

TTFM Findings

PI:	10.5	Insufficiency:	45.8%
		Mean flow without proximal snare:	−8.0 mL/min

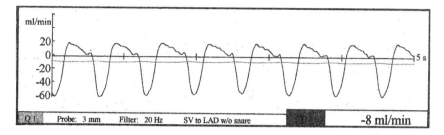

Figure 30. SVG → LAD without snare, mean flow − 8.0 mL/min.

Comment

At first glance, it appeared that there was a diastolic curve without any systolic spike that would indicate graft patency. However, the insufficiency was extremely high, PI was above normal (>5), and mean flow was expressed as a negative value (−8 mL/min). Note that the line denoting mean flow is below the zero flow line. The distal LIMA was still intact at this point. On the basis of these findings, a bulldog was placed on the LIMA distally to the LIMA-SVG anastomosis. The TTFM findings were as follows:

PI: 1.8   Insufficiency: 0.0%
       Mean flow with
          proximal snare: 17.6 mL/min

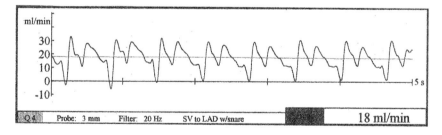

Figure 31. SVG → LAD with snare, mean flow 17.6 mL/min.

TTFM Findings (continued)

PI: 2.4   Insufficiency: 4.1%
       Mean flow without
          proximal snare: 39.1 mL/min

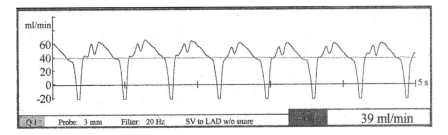

Figure 32. SVG → LAD without snare, mean flow 39.1 mL/min.

Comment

A typical LIMA to the LAD flow pattern is shown with the bulldog placed on the distal LIMA. PI values were normal in both readings with and without snare. Insufficiency was acceptable and greatly reduced from the first reading. Mean flow was adequate with and without snare. TTFM findings were improved after occluding the distal LIMA. In this case TTFM was successful in diagnosing a "steal syndrome" from the distal LIMA.

Patient Outcome

JB did not require graft revision; however, due to the data from the TTFM showing documented "steal syndrome," we did ligate his distal LIMA. The patient remained postoperatively stable. Before discharge, a transthoracic Doppler study confirmed a diastolic flow pattern in the LIMA. At 4-month follow-up, the patient was free from angina or SOB.

Case #8

Clinical History

EP is an 84-year-old female with a 6-month history of angina. A diagnosis of MI was made. Comorbidities included:

♦ HTN

Ventriculography

Left ventriculogram showed hypokinesis of the LV with an EF% of 50%.

Angiographic Findings

The LM coronary artery showed an 80% stenosis in the mid-portion. The LAD showed a 90% stenosis in the proximal portion. The intermediate branch had a 90% stenosis in its proximal portion. The RCA and CX were normal.

Operation

The patient underwent OPCABG via median sternotomy. The bypasses were performed as follows:

♦ SVG → LAD
♦ SVG → OM1

The SVG was anastomosed to a 1.5-mm LAD. A 2.5-mm OM1 was bypassed with SVG. TTFM findings for the SVG → OM1 were within normal limits. Findings in the LAD graft were as follows:

PI: 58.4   Insufficiency: 74.3%
              Mean flow with
              proximal snare: 0.5 mL/min

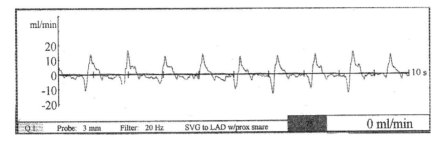

Figure 33. SVG → LAD with snare, mean flow 0.5 mL/min.

TTFM Findings (continued)

PI: 2.0   Insufficiency: 0.2%
                  Mean flow without
                    proximal snare: 10.9 mL/min

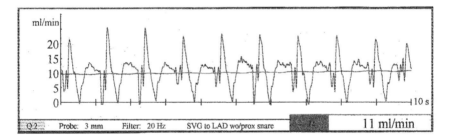

Figure 34. SVG → LAD without snare, mean flow 10.9 mL/min.

Comment

In the first measurement with proximal snare, there was evidence of a problem. The curve demonstrated a sharp systolic spike, and no diastolic flow. PI and insufficiency were very elevated. The mean flow was zero. Yet when the snare was removed, the TTFM values were within normal limits, and the curve demonstrated a typical rounded diastolic flow pattern, with a small diastolic spike. The fact that there was mean flow of 11 mL/min without snare indicates that this flow was probably all retrograde, suggesting an occlusion at the toe of the anastomosis. The LAD anastomosis was revised and explored. A tight lesion on the native coronary distal to the arteriotomy was discovered after passing a probe. A longer arteriotomy was performed and a new anastomosis was done with the following TTFM findings.

TTFM Findings

PI: 1.8   Insufficiency: 0.5%
                Mean flow with
                   proximal snare: 9.4 mL/min

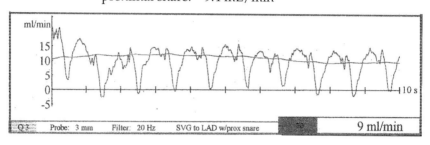

Figure 35. SVG → LAD with snare, mean flow 9.4 mL/min.

TTFM Findings (continued)

PI: 1.4   Insufficiency: 0.0%
                Mean flow without
                   proximal snare: 23.6 mL/min

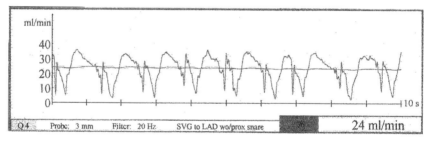

Figure 36. SVG → LAD without snare, mean flow 23.6 mL/min.

Comment

In flow measurements both with and without snare, there was clearly a diastolic flow pattern without a systolic spike. TTFM values were within normal limits. PI and insufficiency were low and, although mean flow value was low with snare, the curve and PI value indicated graft patency. It is important, when evaluating TTFM findings, that all indices are taken into account. The mean flow value without snare fell within the range for a 1.5-mm LAD (35 mL/min ± 15 mL/min).

Patient Outcome

Patient was discharged after 5 days. She has remained clinically stable. At 3-month follow-up, she was symptom free.

Case #9

Clinical History

DM is a 69-year-old white male with chronic atrial fibrillation and mild dyspnea on exertion. The patient's cormorbidities included:

- Chronic atrial fibrillation
- Hypercholesterolemia

Ventriculography

Left ventriculogram showed hypokinesis with an EF of 50%.

Angiography

The LAD had a 50% ostial lesion as well as a 90% lesion of the LAD after the origin of the first diagonal. The DIAG had an 80% stenosis at its origin. The bypasses were performed as follows:

- LIMA → LAD
- SVG→ DIAG

Operation

The patient underwent OPCAB via median sternotomy. The LIMA was anastomosed to a 2.0-mm LAD using a 7.0 Prolene continuous suture. The SVG was anastomosed to a 1.5-mm DIAG using a 7.0 Prolene continuous suture. The TTFM findings for the SVG → DIAG were within normal limits.

TTFM Findings

PI: 3.5   Insufficiency: 6.0%
                Mean flow with
                    proximal snare: 10.7 mL/min

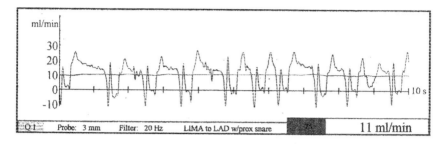

Figure 37. LIMA → LAD with snare, mean flow 10.7 mL/min.

TTFM Findings (continued)

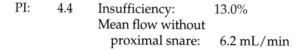

PI: 4.4   Insufficiency: 13.0%
                Mean flow without
                  proximal snare: 6.2 mL/min

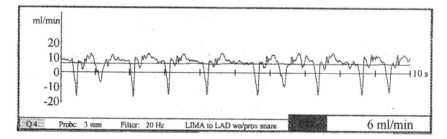

Figure 38. LIMA → LAD without snare, mean flow 6.2 mL/min.

Comment

In both curves there was good diastolic flow patterns, with no systolic spikes. The flow, without proximal snare, was low (6 mL/min). PIs fell within the normal range (<5). After applying the snare, the curve remained unchanged, PIs were still within the normal range, and actual flow was mildly increased (11 mL/min).

The actual flow appeared to be low for a 2-mm LAD. This graft was measured repeatedly with the same results. In spite of that, the surgeon decided not to revise the graft because the remaining TTFM data (PI values and flow pattern) were suggestive for a patent anastomosis. At inspection of the anastomotic site, a hematoma, caused by the stabilizer foot, was noted. It was thought that perhaps the hematoma was compressing the lateral wall of the LAD. After having "released" the hematoma with local dissection, flow measurements were performed again.

TTFM Findings

PI: 2.4   Insufficiency: 3.7%
Mean flow without
proximal snare: 32.0 mL/min

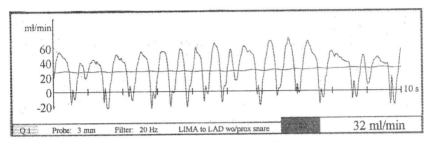

Figure 39. LIMA → LAD without snare, mean flow 32.0 mL/min.

Comment

The TTFM data remained as they were before, within normal limits; however, the mean flow increased to 32 mL/min. This is an important point, because the TTFM indicated a functioning graft with a patent anastomosis, but a suspiciously low flow for a 2.0-mm LAD. This graft and its anastomosis were functioning, yet flow was still impeded. It is important to note that all criteria need to be considered when measuring flow.

Characteristics of Patent Grafts

Case #10

Clinical History

MB is a 67-year-old man with no history of MI, and a positive stress test. Comorbidities included:

♦ Hypercholesterolemia
♦ Peripheral vascular disease (PVD)

Ventriculography

The EF was 35%, with inferior basal akinesis.

Angiographic Findings

The LM was patent. The LAD showed a proximal 75% narrowing just after a medium sized D1 artery. The RCA was occluded with diffused calcifications.

Operation

The patient underwent OPCAB via median sternotomy. The following graft was performed:

♦ LIMA→ LAD

The LAD had a 2.0-mm lumen, and the anastomosis was performed using 7.0 Prolene running suture.

TTFM Findings

PI: 1.7   Insufficiency: 0.7%
              Mean flow with
                 proximal snare: 35.6 mL/min

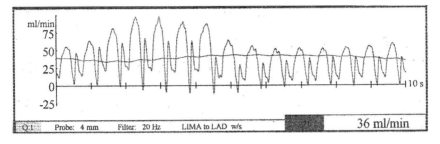

Figure 40. LIMA → LAD with snare, mean flow 35.6 mL/min.

TTFM Findings (continued)

PI: 3.1   Insufficiency: 4.8%
              Mean flow without
                  proximal snare: 29.4 mL/min

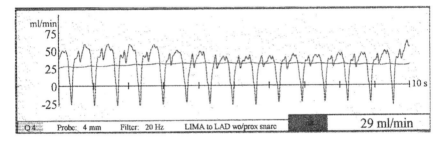

Figure 41. LIMA → LAD without snare, mean flow 29.4 mL/min.

These are typical LIMA → LAD flow curves, with and without snare. There was a small systolic spike, followed by a much larger diastolic curve. There was minimal insufficiency, and PIs were within normal limits (<5.0). In this particular type of graft, mean flow is frequently found to be equal to 30 mL/min ± 15 mL/min. The flow may go down when the snare is taken off due to competition from the native vessel. Likewise, it may go up when the snare is applied.

Patient Outcome

MB had normal TTFM findings for a LIMA → LAD. There were no elevations of CPK(MB) postoperatively. He was discharged without complications in stable condition. He started phase 2 cardiac rehab 2 weeks after discharge. The patient did not follow up at 3 months.

Case #11

Clinical History

RC is a 55-year-old white male with a history of chest pain and SOB. Family history was positive for CAD.

Ventriculography

Left ventricular EF was 50–55%.

Angiographic Findings

The LAD was a moderate sized vessel, with a long 95% lesion in its mid-portion. The RCA was a moderate to large vessel. There were diffuse irregularities throughout its course.

Operation

The patient underwent OPCABG via median sternotomy. Bypasses were performed as follows:

♦ LIMA → LAD
♦ RIMA → RCA

The RCA was a 3-mm vessel. A 7.0 Prolene running suture was used for the distal anastomosis. The flow curves demonstrate a typical RIMA → RCA graft.

TTFM Findings

PI: 1.1   Insufficiency: 0.0%
                  Mean flow with
                      proximal snare: 65.0 mL/min

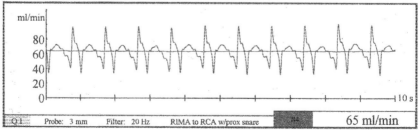

Figure 42. RIMA → RCA with snare, mean flow 65.0 mL/min.

TTFM Findings (continued)

PI: 1.3   Insufficiency: 0.0%
                Mean flow without
                   proximal snare: 45.2 mL/min

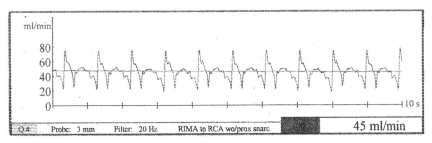

Figure 43. RIMA → RCA without snare, mean flow 45.2 mL/min.

Comment

It is very common for a graft to the RCA to have a more prominent systolic curve, along with a good quality diastolic flow curve. In contrast to the other coronary branches, flow in the RCA takes place also during systole. These curves were satisfactory. There was no insufficiency, the PIs were low, and flows were in the range for a 3-mm vessel. Again, it is noted that the flow decreases when the snare is removed due to competition from the native vessel.

Patient Outcome

TTFM findings were normal. The patient had no elevations of CPK(MB) postoperatively. The patient was discharged without complications, and in stable condition. At his 3-month follow-up, he was doing well with no complaints. He has begun his cardiac rehabilitation.

Case #12

Clinical History

EP is a 64-year-old white male, who denied any history of MI. The patient had recent onset of chest pressure radiating to both shoulders. Medical history was positive for hypothyroidism. Family history was positive for CAD. Comorbidities included cigarette smoking.

Ventriculography

The EF% was 50%, with mild basal hypokinesia.

Angiographic Findings

The LAD had severe disease with 95% proximal stenosis and a second subocclusive distal lesion. The DIAG branch was similarly affected with a very critical 95% stenosis.

Operation

The patient underwent OPCABG via median sternotomy. Bypasses performed were as follows:

- LIMA → LAD
- SVG → DIAG

DIAG had a lumen of 1.5 mm. A 7.0 Prolene running suture was used. Both grafts demonstrated good flow by TTFM.

TTFM Findings

The following TTFM findings were typical for a SVG → DIAG bypass:

PI: 2.8   Insufficiency: 4.6%
                Mean flow with
                   proximal snare: 21.1 mL/min

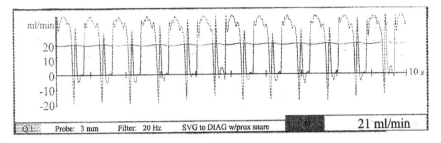

Figure 44. SVG → DIAG with snare, mean flow 21.1 mL/min.

TTFM Findings (continued)

PI: 2.9   Insufficiency: 5.3%
               Mean flow without
                  proximal snare: 13.9 mL/min

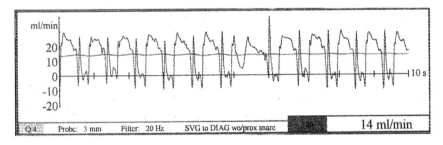

Figure 45. SVG → DIAG without snare, mean flow 13.9 mL/min.

The TTFM curve was mainly diastolic with an almost flat peak, followed by a systolic spike. As is common, the flow was higher with the snare on, and dropped after the snare was off due to competition from the native vessel. PIs were within normal limits, and insufficiency was minimal.

Patient Outcome

EP had normal TTFM findings in both bypasses. There were no complications. He was discharged in stable condition. At the 3-month follow-up, he was without complaints, and had a normal stress test postoperatively.

Case #13

Clinical History

NS is a 56-year-old-white male with no previous medical history. Past surgical history was negative. The patient's risk factors included:

♦ Smoking history
♦ Hypertension

Ventriculography

The EF% was 45%, with inferobasal akinesia.

Angiographic Findings

The LAD was 95% stenosed after the D1. Both D1 and D2 were 95% narrowed. There was diffuse disease throughout the LAD. The CX was occluded prior to the OM1. There was peripheral flow to the OM1 and OM2 via collaterals. The RCA was occluded at the origin. The PDA and posterolateral (PLA) branch filled via collaterals from the left.

Operation

The patient underwent OPCABG via median sternotomy. The bypasses were performed as follows:

♦ LIMA → DIAG
♦ SVG → LAD
♦ SVG → OM1

The SVG was anastomosed to a 2.0-mm OM1 using a 7.0 Prolene running suture. All 3 grafts demonstrated good flow curves via TTFM.

TTFM Findings

The following TTFM findings were typical for SVG → OM1:

PI: 1.9 Insufficiency: 0.0%
Mean flow with
proximal snare: 75.8 mL/min

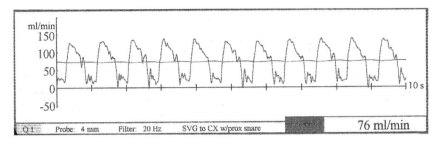

Figure 46. SVG → OM1 with snare, mean flow 75.8 mL/min.

TTFM Findings (continued)

PI: 1.8   Insufficiency: 0.0%
       Mean flow without
           proximal snare: 74.6 mL/min

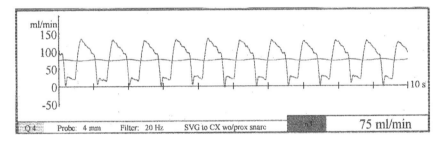

Figure 47. SVG → OM1 without snare, mean flow 74.6 mL/min.

Both curves with and without snare showed the round diastolic pattern that peaks and then slopes down. A slight systolic curve may or may not show up. Low PIs, no insufficiency, and high mean flow exhibit all the qualities of good grafts.

Patient Outcome

NS had normal TTFM findings on all of his bypasses. The purpose of including this patient was to demonstrate a typical SVG → OM1. The patient was discharged without complications, and in stable condition. The patient had a follow-up angiogram confirming patency of all 3 bypasses.

Case #14

Clinical History

WB is a 76-year-old white male with a 3-week history of chest pain and SOB. Comorbidities included:

♦ Previous CABG
♦ PVD

Ventriculography

The EF% was 53%.

Angiographic Findings

The LIMA graft to the D1 and LAD was patent. The RCA showed a 95% stenosis at the origin.

Operation

The patient underwent OPCABG via lower partial sternotomy. One bypass was performed as follows:

♦ Composite graft RGEA/SVG → RCA

The RGEA composite graft was anastomosed to a 1.5-mm PDA using a 7.0 Prolene running suture.

TTFM Findings

PI: 2.6   Insufficiency: 4.1%
            Mean flow with
              proximal snare: 19.0 mL/min

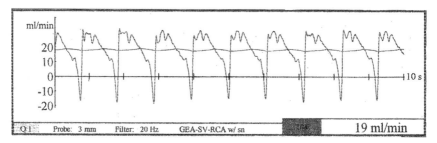

Figure 48. RGEA → SVG → RCA with snare, mean flow 19.0 mL/min.

TTFM Findings (continued)

PI: 3.5   Insufficiency: 2.8%
                Mean flow without
                    proximal snare: 5.7 mL/min

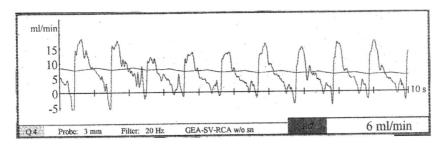

Figure 49. RGEA → SVG → RCA without snare, mean flow 5.7 m/min.

Comment

A very good diastolic flow pattern was demonstrated in both curves. Typical competition from the native vessel was also seen with a lower flow value (6 mL/min) when the snare was removed. The PI showed a normal value (<5). There was minimal insufficiency. On the basis of these findings, the graft was determined to be patent.

Patient Outcome

One year after surgery, the patient was admitted for a pacemaker implant. He was restudied with Doppler and angiogram. The RGEA was patent at both Doppler and angiography.

Index